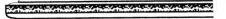

Peter A. Lichtenberg, Ph.

M000288753

Mental Health Practice in Geriatric Health Care Settings

Pre-publication
REVIEWS,
COMMENTARIES,
EVALUATIONS . . .

"**D**r. Lichtenberg has written an ambitious work that spans important areas of geriatric health care. Much of the book is a tour de force of Dr. Lichtenberg's impressive research program into neuropsychological aspects of geriatric rehabilitation. In addition to reviewing clinical research in the areas of depression, dementia, and alcohol abuse, he offers the reader case examples and valuable, practical recommendations for day-to-day clinical care. This book will be a valuable resource for psychologists and other clinicians who treat older adults."

Stephen Rapp, PhD
Associate Professor in Psychiatry/
Chief of Psychology,
Bowman Gray School of Medicine,
Wake Forest University,
Winston-Salem, NC

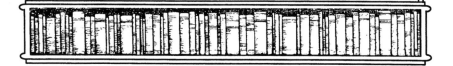

More pre-publication
REVIEWS, COMMENTARIES, EVALUATIONS . . .

"Lichtenberg's book, *Mental Health Practice in Geriatric Health Care Settings*, provides a plethora of useful information for mental health practitioners, medical personnel, and the designers of integrated delivery systems of health care for older adults. He describes new research findings from studies of an elderly urban population in a rehabilitation setting in addition to summarizing the findings that demonstrate the relationship between health outcomes and cognitive status and mood.

Even the most experienced geropsychologist will learn practical clinical tips for neuropsychological assessment approaches and treatment protocols for frail older adults. This book pushes the field of geriatric behavioral health care one giant step ahead by describing health outcome data, treatment protocols for depression, and case examples of how neuropsychological data can be implemented into cost-saving treatment planning."

Paula E. Hartman-Stein, PhD
Founder, Center for Healthy Aging;
Senior Fellow, Institute
for Life-Span Development
and Gerontology,
University of Akron

"This book provides a thorough review of the research pertinent to the mental health of older patients suffering physical health problems. It is an excellent source of information about and evaluation of various assessment instruments for use with older people.

The chapter on depression in geriatric health outcomes should be especially helpful to the mental health professional. It provides methods for assessing depression and an excellent protocol for the treatment of depression in older medical patients.

The chapters on the assessment of cognition and Alzheimer's disease also provide a review of the most recent research that will be useful to the practitioner.

The chapters on the changes taking place in health care in general, and geriatric health care practice in particular, give a useful overview of the situation as it exists at the present time.

This book should be a useful addition to the library of any psychologist practicing with older medical patients."

Clifford H. Swensen, PhD
Professor of Psychology,
Purdue University

"Lichtenberg has assembled an extensive composite of material on geriatric mental health care. This book is a unique collection of current empirical studies, underlying theoretical perspectives, normative data, and case examples. Each chapter provides meaningful clinical implications and key references. A comprehensive examination of the most central issues in clinical geropsychology is covered, including the complex relationship between physical and mental health, the impact of normal aging and disease on cognitive functioning, geriatric neuropsychological assessment, and the evaluation and treatment of depression and alcohol abuse. It is an exceptional package of information about the most common problems that psychologists and mental health providers encounter in older adults.

Lichtenberg is a seasoned clinical geropsychologist who draws on his wealth of experience to educate clinicians who are new to geriatrics and to update experienced practitioners in the field. The book is also an invaluable contribution for gerontologists who work with minority, urban elders—we finally have data and perspectives based on this vast population and no longer have to rely on knowledge exclusively drawn from white, middle-class, well-educated older adults.

As a researcher, clinical supervisor, and psychologist who consults in long-term care, I highly recommend this book because it provides the fundamental tools that all gerontologists must have to deliver competent mental health services in health care facilities. The comprehensive information compiled in this single source is an invaluable asset to all geriatric mental health providers."

Margaret P. Norris, PhD
Associate Professor,
Texas A&M University

"Drawing upon his extensive experience at a large urban medical center, Peter Lichtenberg presents a clearly written summary of pertinent mental health issues affecting geriatric medical and rehabilitation patients. He offers recent literature, substantive data, and practical suggestions to assist the clinician and clinical researcher. Dr. Lichtenberg always keeps daily functioning and independence as the most important outcomes, as they should be in geriatrics."

Bryan Kemp, PhD
Director, Rehabilitation Research
and Training Center on Aging,
Rancho Los Amigos Medical Center,
Downey, CA

Mental Health Practice in Geriatric Health Care Settings

HAWORTH Aging, Psychology, and Mental Health
T. L. Brink, PhD
Senior Editor

A Guide to Psychological Practice in Geriatric Long-Term Care
by Peter A. Lichtenberg

Mental Health Practice in Geriatric Health Care Settings
by Peter A. Lichtenberg

Mental Health Practice in Geriatric Health Care Settings

Peter A. Lichtenberg, PhD, ABPP

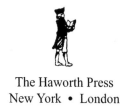

The Haworth Press
New York • London

The Haworth Press, Inc., 10 Alice Street, Binghamton, NY 13904-1580

Cover design by Marylouise E. Doyle.

Library of Congress Cataloging-in-Publication Data

Lichtenberg, Peter A.
    Mental health practice in geriatric health care settings / Peter A. Lichtenberg.
        p.   cm.
    Includes bibliographical references (p.   ).
    ISBN 0-7890-0435-6 (alk. paper).
    1. Geriatric psychiatry. 2. Aged—Mental health. I. Title.
RC451.4.A5L53 1997
618.97'689—dc21
                                                                        97-21734
                                                                        CIP

To the very special ladies who have graced my life: Bertha Russell, Bertha Lichtenberg, Elsa Russell Lichtenberg, Rebecca Classen Lichtenberg, Emily Katherine Lichtenberg, and Susan Ellen MacNeill, and to my dad, Philip Lichtenberg

ABOUT THE AUTHOR

Peter A. Lichtenberg, PhD, ABPP, is Associate Professor of Physical Medicine and Rehabilitation at Wayne State University School of Medicine and Associate Director of Rehabilitation Psychology and Neuropsychology at the Rehabilitation Institute of Michigan. He received his PhD in clinical psychology from Purdue University, where he also minored in aging. He completed specialty internship training in clinical geropsychology at the Gainesville Veterans Affairs Medical Center and his postdoctoral training in geriatric neuropsychology at the University of Virginia Medical School, where he served on the faculty from 1987 to 1990. He is author of *A Guide to Psychological Practice in Geriatric Long-Term Care* (The Haworth Press, 1993) and Chief Editor for the book series Advances in Medical Psychotherapy. Dr. Lichtenberg has written more than seventy scientific papers in the areas of clinical geropsychology and geriatric neuropsychology.

CONTENTS

Foreword

Alvin Toffler (1970) describes "future shock" as "the shattering stress and disorientation that we induce in individuals by subjecting them to too much change in too short a time." Clinicians are aware of this future shock and the challenges inherent in the volatile health care environment, the harsh new economic realities, and the advancing age of our treatment populations. Now more than ever, the clinician must be armed with sufficient empirical data to meet the needs of our rapidly expanding geriatric patient groups. Normative studies are critical to our understanding of important social and psychological factors that affect outcome, and we must place new emphasis on clinical and experimental programs of research that stress psychosocial services for our elderly. This melding of science and practice is the focus of *Mental Health Practice in Geriatric Health Care Settings.*

Dr. Lichtenberg has captured the essence of the struggle to understand the comorbidity between medical and mental health problems in this elderly population. He examines the influences of depression, cognitive slippage, substance abuse, medication toxicity, and degenerative neurologic processes on outcomes such as competence in activities of daily living and morbidity/mortality. The author uses his own large subject normative study (The Normative Studies Research Project Battery) as a data anchor or reference point to determine the influence of cognitive, emotional, neurologic, and social factors in *real* clinical cases. This book specifically focuses on the detection and treatment of depression, cognitive impairment, and alcohol abuse using a behavioral approach and offering impairment-based, sequential intervention techniques. The last two chapters delineate emerging areas in geriatric health care such as competency evaluations, treatment of pain and anxiety, and survival strategies for all who are concerned by the disincentives for offering quality care to this often neglected population.

Mental Health Practice in Geriatric Health Care Settings sensitizes us to the psychological factors and problems that are quite common—yet often go undetected—in the elderly. The author provides us with the methodologies for accurate detection of these problems and delineates successful cost-effective intervention strategies that can easily supplement traditional medical therapies.

Jeffrey T. Barth, PhD, ABPP

Acknowledgments

I am most grateful to Jeff Barth and Jeff Dwyer. Jeff Barth has given me monumental support throughout this project and throughout my career. Jeff Dwyer spent countless hours helping me think through this book, editing drafts of the manuscript, and encouraging me to continue. I am very grateful to Lise Youngblade whose technical support and encouragement were so very helpful. I am indebted to a number of other colleagues who helped edit my work: Kathleen Sitley Brown, Bernice Marcopulos, Phil Fastenau, Susan MacNeill, Bob Guenther, and Michael Kimbarow. I thank my parents for their strong support, and John Pepper for his loving friendship.

Introduction

The Links Between Physical and Mental Health

Mental health practitioners often bemoan the fact that older adults utilize mental health services less than do younger adults. It has long been known, however, that older adults do not separate their mental health symptoms from their physical symptoms (Brody, Kleban, and Moles, 1983). Indeed, primary care physicians are routinely confided in by their older patients regarding patients' mental health symptoms. This phenomenon was termed the "inseparability of mental and physical health problems" by Patricia Parmelee and her colleagues at a symposium during the 1996 Gerontological Society of America's annual meeting. Unfortunately for patients, physicians are not well trained in the assessment and treatment of psychosocial problems. Although physicians are required in the history and physical examination to document current social and psychological functioning of the patient, this is typically undertaken in a cursory manner. Physicians in both primary care and medical rehabilitation practices fail to detect routine problems such as depression in well over three-quarters of their cases (Lichtenberg et al., 1993; Rapp, Parisi, and Walsh, 1988; Schuckit et al., 1980). Patients, in turn, do not get the treatment they need. The lack of physician training, combined with the increasing evidence that psychosocial factors are very strong influences on health outcomes, provide great challenges and opportunities for mental health practitioners. The objective of this book is to help mental health practitioners meet these challenges and seize opportunities in health care. Three themes will be incorporated into each of the major ideas presented in this book: first, geriatric patients' needs are best served through multidisciplinary practice; second, given the changing health care environment in the United States, empirical support must be provided for all new mental health practices; and third, this book will focus on a unique population—urban elderly from a midwestern city.

Given the increasing patient care demands upon physicians, the best way to address mental health problems is through multidisciplinary linkages. *Multidisciplinarity* refers to a number of health professionals from different disciplines working with the same patient. In this way it is hoped that the patient's physical, psychological, and social needs will all be identified and treated. Multidisciplinary teams collaborate through an exchange of information and through consultation. A mental health practitioner might, therefore, inform a physician as to how depression or anxiety might be affecting adherence to a treatment regimen. *Interdisciplinarity* refers to close collaboration between team members, where more than one discipline works on the same goal. In interdisciplinary practice, a nurse and occupational therapist, for example, might adopt the same treatment plan to work on a patient's grooming and bathing. Due to both time constraints and to a lack of knowledge about other disciplines, most health care teams work together in a cursory multidisciplinary fashion (Lichtenberg, 1994).

Mental health practitioners in health care settings may be underutilized or utilized inappropriately, particularly because other team members lack an understanding of how psychosocial issues fit into health care treatment and outcomes. Specific methods of how mental health practitioners can educate their medical colleagues in regard to the effects of psychosocial problems on health will be provided. In addition, methods to improve treatment through multi- and interdisciplinary approaches will be presented. One of the major themes of this book then will be to describe ways that mental health practitioners can effectively integrate themselves into multidisciplinary efforts.

A second underlying theme of this book will be the use of empirical and statistical data to support the role of mental health practitioners in health care settings. Demonstrating the importance of psychosocial variables through empirical and statistical data is now an essential component for mental health practitioners to survive in health care settings. Whereas five to ten years ago data was not an essential element in health care, now administrators from operations, quality assurance, and finance, as well as clinical directors from all departments, are trained to collect and analyze basic data. How and why did this transformation take place? The use of data in hospital systems coincided with the implementation nationwide of systemic improvement efforts known as Continuous Improvement or Total Quality Management (Hertz, 1989). These efforts were aimed at improving hospital processes through interdisciplinary teams (which included patients input as well), and through the use of empirical evaluation of stated goals. Having their roots in the automotive industry, these improvement processes were aimed at improving inefficiencies that were caused by poor communication and integration between departments.

The quality improvement processes changed the way programs are viewed. Administrators have gained confidence and savvy in viewing data, and practitioners are being forced to catch up. A proposal for a program now must include preliminary data and statistical analyses (or at least a plan for these) before any administrator will evaluate the merits of the proposal. In order for mental health practitioners to broaden their role in health care settings, then, they are going to need data that support their aims. This book will present clinically relevant data in order to give clinicians some of the empirical and statistical material they will need. This represents a change in how books are typically written for clinicians. In writing the book *A Guide to Psychological Practice in Long-Term Care,* I emphasized ideas and case examples and used data sparingly. The present volume will attempt to present ideas, cases, and data in a more equal fashion.

The geographical and medical settings that provided the context for this book are important to delineate. The health system that served as the primary base for this material is in central city Detroit. This area, similar to other cities, has a larger prevalence of older adults than do suburban areas, and a majority of the residents in this area are minorities and poor. Hirshorn (1993) reported on the population in central Detroit. Seventy-five percent of the population over age 60 were African Americans, 22 percent were whites, and all other minority groups made up less than 1 percent each. Fifty-nine percent of the population were females and 41 percent were males.

Men tended to be concentrated in the 60 to 74 age group. Two-thirds of the residents in this area had an annual household income of $10,000 or less, and 29 percent of these residents had an annual income of $5,000 or less. Over 86 percent of all residents in senior housing had their rents subsidized by the government. Over half of the older community residents had lived in their neighborhoods for 16 or more years. For a multitude of reasons, the work on mental health in health care settings has often failed to include patients from the cities. Thus, information on geriatric neuropsychology, depression, and substance abuse in urban elderly, for example, is sorely lacking. This book drew its data from a central city Detroit hospital. Ninety percent of the hospital's geriatric patients came from the central city region, and as such, this volume can serve to present new information on urban elderly, the majority of whom are African Americans.

A medical-rehabilitation hospital served as the site for the work that was undertaken. Medical rehabilitation has its roots in treating war wounds earlier in the twentieth century, and then as a primary treatment for functional gains in those with polio. More recently, rehabilitation has been focused upon helping survivors of traumatic brain and spinal cord injuries resume active and productive lives. Stroke rehabilitation has also been a mainstay of medical rehabilitation, and because older adults are the most likely to experience strokes, geriatric patients have been served in medical rehabilitation for decades. Nevertheless, it has only been in the past decade that adults over age 60 have made up the largest percentage of medical rehabilitation settings (Lichtenberg and Rosenthal, 1994).

To qualify for medical rehabilitation, older adults have to experience a primary rehabilitation diagnosis and secondary medical diseases that complicate recovery from the primary problem. Common primary diagnoses in medical rehabilitation include stroke, orthopedic injuries, lower extremity amputations due to diabetes, lower extremity fractures, and muscular weakness. Blood pressure and heart and systemic diseases such as diabetes and arthritis are common secondary diagnoses.

Older adults in medical rehabilitation stay in the rehabilitation hospital from 10 to 20 days. Medical rehabilitation, for older adults, has as its focus functional improvements and optimal independence. To accomplish this, patients undertake at least three hours of therapy per day, including what they need in physical, occupational, speech, social work, and psychological services. Much of the focus is on safe transfers, from the bed to a chair for example, and other activities of daily living (ADLs) such as using adaptive devices to help bathe or dress oneself, and learning how to ambulate with a walker or cane. The completion of a medical rehabilitation program is a strenuous task for older adults who are made frail by many systemic diseases. Motivation, perseverance, and mental flexibility are all required for the patient to be successful.

Patients in the Rehabilitation Institute of Michigan, which services the inner city of Detroit, had primary medical rehabilitation diagnoses consistent with other medical rehabilitation programs. Cerebral dysfunction represented the highest percentage of primary diagnoses, and this included strokes. Muscular weakness represented the second most prevalent primary diagnosis, and fractures of the lower extremity represented the third largest primary diagnosis. Hypertension and diabetes represented the most common secondary diagnosis, and over 60 percent of patients in our facility were hypertensive, while 35 percent were diagnosed with diabetes. Congestive heart failure, coronary artery disease, and peripheral vascular disease were the other most common secondary diagnoses.

Each chapter in this book will reflect the three underlying themes of multidisciplinarity, empirical and statistical investigation, and the focus upon the urban elderly. In addition, the major objective of this book is to provide clinicians with new understandings and new assessment and treatment knowledge to use in their practice. Finally, this book endeavors to provide clinicians with information about emerging trends in the field, and effective strategies for practice in health care settings.

Chapter 1

Overview

Geriatric health care settings represent an optimal place for mental health professionals to practice. The term "comorbidity" refers to the co-occurrence of diseases. In this chapter, we will review the comorbidity of medical and psychosocial problems—that is, whether psychosocial problems are common in medical rehabilitation patients—and whether there are enough psychosocial problems in geriatric medical patients for them to be given treatment consideration by hospitals. A second type of comorbidity, that of the co-occurrence of two or more psychosocial problems, will also be explored later in this chapter. Comorbid problems such as dementia, delirium, depression, and substance abuse and their occurrence in older medical patients were recently studied by our research group.

PHYSICAL DISEASES AND FUNCTIONAL OUTCOME IN 1,000 OLDER URBAN MEDICAL PATIENTS

Our five-year project has led to the study of over 1,000 consecutive admissions of patients ages 60 to 103 years to a geriatric rehabilitation unit for older adults in the Rehabilitation Institute of Michigan, described earlier. This sample, which was studied for various purposes throughout the five years, provides the basis of many of the mental health assessment and treatment practices described in this book. The sample characteristics will be discussed, and the comorbidity of physical and mental health problems illustrated. The 1,000-patient sample consisted of 67 percent African Americans and 33 percent white (Latino, Arab-American, and Asian patients were eliminated due to small numbers). Two-thirds of the sample were women.

Hanks and Lichtenberg (1996) investigated the comorbidities for a variety of physical, functional, psychological, and social variables by dividing the patients into four groups by decades: ages 60 to 69 (n = 131), 70 to 79 (n = 363), 80 to 89 (n = 263), and 90 to 103 (n = 55). The racial makeup of the groups was no different across the different ages, but not surprisingly, the oldest decades were made up of significantly more women than was the youngest decade. Principal diagnoses also differed for the age groups. Stroke was a much more common primary diagnosis among the younger groups, whereas hip fractures from falls were more common in the older groups. Mean education ranged from 10.55 years for the youngest group to 8.56 years in the oldest group, but these differences were not statistically significant (see Table 1.1).

Comorbid physical disease was measured by Charlson and colleagues' (1987) index of comorbidity. This measure was later validated in our sample (see the 1996 Moore and Lichtenberg study summarized in Chapter 2). An interesting and startling pattern emerged. Contrary to our expectations, the younger patients exhibited significantly worse comorbid illness. The younger adult patients actually suffered from more diseases and from more serious comorbid diseases than did the oldest patients. This sample of younger patients represented an extremely ill sample relative to the base rates of problems in community samples in this age group.

Measures of psychological variables helped to demonstrate this. Whereas the base rate of significant cognitive dysfunction in the community was 15 percent for those ages 60 to 79 (Evans et al., 1989), the prevalence of cognitive dysfunction in our sample for these ages was 40 percent. In our sample, the prevalence of depression was 35 percent compared to community estimates of 15 percent (Blazer, Hughes, and George, 1987). Finally, whereas alcohol abuse was estimated to be present in less than 5 percent of the community samples, it was present in 19 percent of our sample ages 60 to 79 years. Clearly, the younger patients, ages 60 to 79 years, represent a significantly impaired population, and a population of inseparable physical and mental health disease. The oldest group, while more representative of the community population ages 80 to 103, also demonstrated significant comorbid physical and mental health problems. Cognitive dysfunction was present in 60 percent

TABLE 1.1. Demographics by Age Group (Mean scores)

	60-69 (n = 131)	70-79 (n = 363)	80-89 (n = 263)	90-103 (n = 55)	Significant Level
Education	10.55	9.82	9.61	8.56	ns
Race					
Black	88 (67%)	228 (63%)	153 (58%)	35 (64%)	ns
White	42 (32%)	135 (37%)	110 (42%)	20 (36%)	
Other	1 (.7%)				
Gender					
Male	57 (44%)	133 (37%)	72 (27%)	19 (35%)	.01
Female	74 (56%)	230 (63%)	191 (73%)	36 (65%)	
Principal Diagnosis					
Cerebral Dysfunction	41 (32%)	83 (23%)	44 (17%)	12 (22%)	.001
Muscular Weakness	65 (50%)	194 (55%)	108 (42%)	20 (36%)	
Fractures	18 (14%)	70 (20%)	100 (39%)	22 (40%)	
Other	5 (4%)	8 (2%)	7 (3%)	1 (2%)	
Length of Stay	17.85	18.22	19.40	18.07	ns
Comorbidity Index	2.92	2.38	2.10	2.09	.001

of our older patients, compared to base rate estimates of 45 percent. Depression and alcohol abuse were present at twice the rate in our sample (27 percent and 8 percent respectively) as compared to base rate estimates.

The groups may represent different populations. It is likely that patients in the younger group (ages 60 to 79) do not survive into the older group. Patients in the older group who were vigorous in their younger years are only now finding themselves in health care settings. The oldest group is made up of those that survive into older age and then become disabled, while the younger group is likely to have a high mortality rate before many of its members reach age 80 and beyond.

The Functional Independence Measure (FIM) was used to measure physical functioning. The FIM is an observer-rated instrument that rates 18 items for patient motor functioning (ambulation and

ADLs) and patient social cognition skills. Each item is rated on a scale from 1 (total dependence) to 7 (total independence). FIM scores are presented for the six areas of handicap: ADLs, bowel and bladder management, communication skills, locomotion skills, mobility, and social cognition. These scales are created by simply adding item totals together.

Physical function and living situations show a linear effect for age, despite the differences in comorbid physical and psychological illness. Functional abilities after medical rehabilitation were significantly better for the younger patients in all categories as compared to the older patients (see Table 1.2). As can be seen in the table, these abilities represent ADL abilities, bowel and bladder functioning, communication skills, locomotion skills, mobility skills, and social cognition skills. Thus, despite the relative severity of illness in the younger group, the group recovered to higher levels of independence than did the older group. As can be seen in Table 1.3, there was a linear relationship between age and the percentage of individuals who were independent in their abilities. Whereas 43 percent of 60 to 69-year-old patients were independent in ADLs upon discharge, for example, only 7 percent of those ages 90 to 103 years were independent. Advanced age and weakness tend to compromise the functional abilities of the oldest patients. Younger patients possess enough strength to demonstrate greater gains during the medical rehabilitation hospitalization.

The relationship between age and living situation was not a straightforward one. While there were no differences across ages in terms of the percentage of patients who lived alone prior to admission to the hospital (40 percent), there were clear age differences at discharge. Whereas 50 percent of the younger patients who were living alone at admission returned to live alone at discharge, only 30 percent of those over age 80 did so. Discharges to nursing homes illustrates this point even more clearly. While only 5 percent of those ages 60 to 69 years were discharged to nursing homes, 18 percent of those ages 80 to 89 years were, and 29 percent of those ages 90 to 103 were discharged to nursing homes. Discharges to a more dependent level of care ranged from 35 percent in the youngest group to 60 percent of the oldest group. Clearly, the oldest group was the most likely to lose independence due to a hospitalization.

TABLE 1.2. Mean FIM Composite Scores by Age Group

	60s	70s	80s	90s +	Significant Level
ADLs					
Admit	26.46	25.17	23.52	21.15	ns
Discharge	31.12	30.58	28.68	25.46	.00001
Bowel and Bladder					
Admit	9.15	8.81	8.33	6.66	.01
Discharge	11.03	10.36	10.02	9.06	.02
Communication					
Admit	11.15	10.61	10.01	8.76	.006
Discharge	11.38	11.13	10.43	9.53	.001
Locomotion					
Admit	4.68	4.40	4.00	3.78	ns
Discharge	7.20	7.09	6.53	5.60	.007
Mobility					
Admit	10.41	9.92	9.37	8.20	ns
Discharge	13.98	14.00	13.29	11.93	.003
Social Cognition					
Admit	15.43	14.77	13.33	11.65	.00001
Discharge	16.03	15.56	14.26	13.07	.00001

The conclusions from these data are important for mental health practitioners in geriatric health care settings. Geriatric medical patients represent a frail group. They are not only suffering from medical disease, but also from loss of physical function, a heightened rate of psychosocial problems, and real losses of independence. Mental health problems are very common concerns for older medical patients and yet have been too often ignored (Hanks and Lichtenberg, 1996). Mental health practitioners must not only demonstrate that these psychosocial problems are abundant, but that these problems are also key factors in health outcomes.

TABLE 1.3. FIM Outcomes by Age Group—Patients Who Scored as Independent versus Dependent

		60s	70s	80s	90s	Signif. Level
ADLs						
Discharge:	I	12 (9%)	19 (5%)	3 (1.2%)	0 (0%)	.00005
	D	117 (91%)	336 (95%)	256 (98.8%)	55 (100%)	
Discharge:	I	55 (43%)	128 (36%)	61 (24%)	4 (7%)	.00001
	D	74 (57%)	227 (64%)	198 (76%)	51 (93%)	
Bowel and Bladder						
Admit:	I	49 (38%)	117 (33%)	71 (27%)	3 (5%)	.003
	D	80 (62%)	238 (67%)	188 (73%)	52 (95%)	
Discharge:	I	84 (65%)	218 (61%)	140 (54%)	18 (33%)	.0001
	D	45 (35%)	137 (39%)	119 (46%)	37 (67%)	
Communication						
Admit:	I	76 (59%)	177 (50%)	103 (40%)	16 (29%)	.00001
	D	53 (41%)	178 (50%)	156 (60%)	39 (71%)	
Discharge:	I	84 (65%)	218 (61%)	130 (50%)	22 (40%)	.0005
	D	45 (35%)	137 (39%)	129 (50%)	33 (60%)	
Locomotion						
Admit:	I	1 (1%)	1 (.3%)	0 (0%)	0 (0%)	ns
	D	128 (99%)	354 (99.7%)	259 (100%)	55 (100%)	
Discharge:	I	8 (6%)	19 (5%)	9 (3%)	1 (2%)	ns
	D	121 (94%)	336 (95%)	250 (97%)	54 (98%)	
Mobility						
Admit:	I	2 (2%)	1 (.3%)	0 (0%)	0 (0%)	ns
	D	127 (98%)	354 (99.7%)	159 (100%)	55 (100%)	
Discharge:	I	33 (26%)	79 (22%)	31 (12%)	0 (0%)	.00001
	D	96 (74%)	276 (78%)	228 (88%)	55 (100%)	
Social Cognition						
Admit:	I	55 (43%)	134 (38%)	55 (21%)	8 (15%)	.00001
	D	74 (57%)	221 (62%)	204 (79%)	47 (85%)	
Discharge:	I	67 (52%)	165 (46%)	84 (32%)	16 (29%)	.00001
	D	62 (48%)	190 (54%)	175 (68%)	39 (71%)	

Note: I = Scored in the Independent Range on the FIM
D = Scored in the Dependent Range on the FIM

The comorbidity among psychosocial problems may be an important factor in the relationship these variables have to health outcomes. The relationship of dementia to delirium will serve to illustrate this concept. Studies on the prevalence of delirium in acute medical settings have demonstrated that dementia patients are several times more likely to be vulnerable to a delirium than are cognitively intact patients.

The relationship between cognition and depression in older adults has also become an area of increased research and discussion during the past decade. The hypothesis that depression may induce dementia or dementialike states (i.e., pseudodementia, Wells, 1979) is a major health concern. Previous studies (see Lichtenberg et al., 1995, for a review) were limited by methodological issues such as small sample sizes, restricted age of participants, and sampling only from extremes of the depression continuum. Lichtenberg and colleagues (1995) improved research in this area by including a sample size of 220, by controlling for demographic variables, by including young-old and old-old participants, and by cross-validating the results. A derivation and cross-validation sample were drawn and matched on age, education, race, and sex. The Geriatric Depression Scale was used to measure depressive symptomatology on a continuum (Yesavage et al., 1983), and the Mattis Dementia Rating Scale (Mattis, 1988) and Wechsler Memory Scale–Revised Logical Memory subtests (Wechsler, 1987) were utilized as cognitive measures. Regression analyses on the derivation and cross-validation samples revealed that depression and cognition had a significant, yet modest relationship. In all, 8 percent of cognition variance was accounted for by depression. Thus, depression appears to influence cognition, but not to the extent that it would mimic a dementia. In the medical setting, the relationship between cognition and depression is a significant one. Cognitive impairment is found more often and in more severe forms in those patients who are depressed as compared to patients who are not depressed.

CLINICAL IMPLICATIONS

The data on comorbidity have important implications for mental health practitioners. The significant relationship between medical illness, disability, and cognitive and psychosocial problems underscores that mental health practice is required in health care settings. Illness and disability are highly related to cognitive impairment, depression, and alcohol abuse, and yet these problems often go overlooked or undetected. The data also revealed that age, education, and gender are important factors in the prevalence of some mental health problems (e.g., cognitive functioning, alcohol abuse), but unrelated to other mental health problems (e.g., depression). Practitioners need to be aware of these influences when assessing for mental health problems in older medical patients.

The significant relationship between cognition and depression also has important implications for clinicians. These data underscore the complications that mental health practitioners face in treatment. Not only is depression a common problem, but depression and cognitive impairment are often problems in the same patient. Thus, clinicians cannot utilize a narrow focus in their initial assessment, and the identification of one mental health problem does not preclude that there will be others. In sum, clinicians are often faced with patients who have multiple physical, medical, and psychosocial problems.

Chapter 2

Influence of Cognition
on Health Outcomes

Mental health variables must be related to health outcomes so that their usefulness can be demonstrated in health care settings. In the previous chapter, we explored how mental health variables commonly coexisted with physical illness variables, and in this chapter we will explore whether one mental health variable, cognition, affects a variety of health outcomes. For the clinician, the data provided here can be used to demonstrate the important linkages that cognition has with health outcomes. Cognition represents a direct measurement of a patient's level of performance, and in the context of a cognitive assessment can represent an indirect measure of a patient's brain functioning. Since cognitive impairment is so common in geriatric health care patients, the main role of cognition as a predictor is its sensitivity to brain dysfunction and decline in cognitive abilities.

Geriatric medical rehabilitation programs may be an optimal setting to study the effects of mental health variables on health outcomes. Patients enter these programs due to a disability such as a stroke or hip fracture that impairs their ability to provide self-care. During the few weeks of rehabilitation, they are taught new techniques to perform activities of daily living (ADLs) and are helped to become physically stronger through intensive physical and occupational therapies. To what extent do cognitive factors predict physical recovery in these older rehabilitation patients? In this chapter, the following will be detailed: a review of the previous literature on the usefulness of cognition in predicting ADL function; a review of studies my colleagues and I conducted on the ability of cognition to predict ADL recovery during medical rehabilitation; a review of the literature on the usefulness of cognition in predicting instrumental activities of daily living (IADL) abilities; a review of our study on the ability of cognition and awareness of deficit in predicting performance-based IADL skills; a review of our study on the ability of cognition to predict which patients (living alone at admission) were able to return home alone at discharge; and a review of our study on the role of cognition in predicting mortality.

THE RELATIONSHIP OF NEUROPSYCHOLOGICAL VARIABLES TO ADL ABILITIES

Although there have not been a tremendous number of studies completed in this area, cognitive abilities have been found to consistently predict ADL abilities in older adults. In 1990, McCue, Rogers and Goldstein investigated the relationship between the Luria Nebraska Neuropsychological Battery (LNNB) and performance on an unpublished assessment of self-care skills (PASS) (McCue, Rogers, and Goldstein, 1990) with a group of elderly neuropsychiatric patients (mean age = 74.52 ± 7.91). Separate multiple regressions were calculated for each of the four domains measured by the PASS. In these, 45 percent of the total variance associated with cognitively oriented self-care tasks was accounted for by the neuropsychological variables. For the physically oriented tasks, only 29 percent of the total variance was accounted for by neuropsychological test performance.

There were several difficulties encountered in interpreting these results. The subjects included in this study were inpatients in an acute psychiatric facility with a variety of diagnoses including dementia, major depressive disorder, or other psychiatric disorders, making generalization to other populations questionable. Of the 58 subjects included in this study, only 5 were male. There is some evidence that males and females perform differently on diverse self-care tasks (Cockburn, Smith, and Wade, 1990). The use of an unpublished measure of functional independence makes it difficult to generalize the results to a clinical setting.

Similar difficulties are encountered with the 1989 study of geriatric patients by Searight et al. This study investigated the relationship of selected tests from the Halstead Reitan Neuropsychological

Battery (HRNB) (Reitan, 1955) to ratings of everyday functioning scale of competence for independent living skills (SCILS) (Searight et al., 1989), an unpublished measure developed for this study. As with the above study by McCue, Rogers, and Goldstein (1990), their use of an unpublished measure of functional independence causes difficulty in translating information from this study to use in clinical work. Results indicated that 33 percent of the variance associated with the SCILS was accounted for in their statistical analysis. The statistical analysis used in this study, however, makes it risky to generalize results. Canonical analysis, unlike multiple regression analysis, maximizes the unique variance between two domains while minimizing the shared variance. As a result, this analysis is particularly subject to sampling bias and requires a minimum subject-to-variables (N:k) ratio of 20 to 1. In addition, given this subjectivity to sampling bias, it is highly desirable to cross validate any results. This study had an N:k ratio of less than 2 to 1, and there was no cross validation reported.

Other studies have targeted the relationship between cognition and ADL abilities for study with specific patient populations such as stroke, geropsychiatric, and Alzheimer's disease patients. Titus et al. (1991) compared perceptual abilities in 25 stroke patients with 25 normal controls, and then correlated these abilities with a performance-based measure of basic ADL tasks. Their sample was relatively young (mean age = 59 years) and well educated (60 percent completed high school or greater). Whereas only one test was related to dressing skills (Visual Discrimination, $r = .47$; $p<.01$), several cognitive tests were related to upper extremity hygiene, eating, and total ADL scores. Correlations ranged from .41 to .57.

Nadler et al. (1993) examined the relationship of the Mattis Dementia Rating Scale (DRS) to self-care skills in 50 psychogeriatric patients. This sample had a mean age of 75 years and a mean educational level of 10.8 years. A performance-based measure of ADL abilities from the occupational therapy field was used. The Dementia Rating Scale total score was significantly related to hygiene skills ($r = .57$). In an extension of this study, Richardson, Nadler, and Malloy (1995) investigated the relationship between several different neuropsychological measures (not including the DRS this time) and ADL abilities. One hundred eight psychogeriatric patients were used as participants, having a mean age of 74 years and a mean educational level of 10.6 years. In this study, cognitive tests were unrelated to ADL abilities.

Other recent research has continued to address the relationship of neuropsychological test data to everyday functioning (Tupper and Cicerone, 1990, 1991). Tuokko and Crockett (1991) reported on a large study of neuropsychological measures, patient self-ratings, and caregiver ratings in normal and demented elderly. They reported that basic self-care skills were the last functions to be affected by dementia. In a medical rehabilitation setting, however, where patients are having to learn new techniques of basic self-care, the relationship of cognition to basic self-care skills may emerge as an important one.

Many of the studies above suffered from methodological weaknesses; shortcomings include reliance on self-report or caregiver report of ADL abilities, small sample sizes, and a failure to measure potential mediator variables such as age and education. Two of our studies on the prediction of ADL functioning in urban older medical rehabilitation patients will be described below.

COGNITION AND ADL RECOVERY IN URBAN MEDICAL REHABILITATION SETTINGS

Investigating the relationship between cognitive abilities and ADL performance in medical rehabilitation patients provides a unique framework. This research paradigm has different characteristics than does investigating the relationship between these variables in a demented sample having no major physical disabilities. First, recovery from a condition such as a hip fracture, stroke, or deconditioning includes a need to compensate as to how to perform self-care skills because the injury has resulted in loss of physical abilities. Adaptive equipment skills and new weight-bearing techniques, for example, must be mastered. Pain and discomfort must be tolerated, and general strengthening exercises must be endured. The relationship between cognitive abilities and self-care skills in older medical rehabilitation patients may be, therefore, a vitally important relationship to study. Self-care demands such as using an adaptive device to help oneself dress requires initiation, sustained attention, and an ability to follow a sequence of unfamiliar behaviors (e.g., obtain device, reach for clothes, hook clothes to device, put clothes on). The same analogy can be made for getting in and out of bed through new transfer techniques. Intact cognitive functioning would appear to be a prerequisite for completing these tasks without supervision or hands-on assistance.

The Functional Independence Measure (FIM) was utilized as the tool to measure ADL skills in the studies described below. The FIM was developed to provide uniform assessment of severity of disability and medical rehabilitation outcome. This seven-level scale of 18 items was designed to be completed by rehabilitation staff according to objective behavioral criteria. A score of one means that a patient needs total assistance to complete the task, and a score of seven means the patient is totally independent for the task. A score of three means that a person needs minimal physical assistance with the task, and a score of five means that the patient needs only supervision (e.g., verbal instructing and reminding) to complete the task. Studies have indicated high levels of reliability and validity for the FIM. Acceptable levels of clinical interrater agreement (correlation coefficients of 0.93 to 0.97) have been reported by Hamilton et al. (1991). In addition, evidence of good concurrent validity with patients recovering from stroke (Wagner and Zuchigna, 1988) and spinal cord injury (Roth et al., 1990), and good predictive validity in multiple sclerosis patients (Granger et al., 1990) have been reported. Finally, researchers have demonstrated the FIM's utility when working with geriatric and demented populations (Wilking, Dowling, and Heeran, 1991). In the present study, the cognitive components of the FIM evaluation were removed and only the ADL components were included (seven items measuring feeding, grooming, bathing, dressing upper and lower body, and transferring to toilet and to tub).

STUDIES TO PREDICT ADLs

Four hundred and twenty-six consecutive admissions to the geriatric rehabilitation unit over a two-and-a-half-year period constituted our next sample. Mean age was 78 years (SD = 7.4), and mean educational level was 9.8 years (SD = 3.5). Mean length of stay was

18.4 days (SD = 7.1), and the mean number of chronic health conditions was 7.5 (SD = 1.5). One-third of these patients were admitted to rehabilitation for a lower extremity fracture, another third for lower extremity weakness or gait disturbance, and the last third due to a central nervous system disorder such as a stroke. Upon admission, the patient's mean functioning for ADLs was in the range of modified dependence, which improved to modified independence upon discharge. Forty-four percent of the patients scored in the cognitively impaired range on the Dementia Rating Scale, and 56 percent scored in the cognitively unimpaired range, using a cutoff score of 123.

Bivariate correlations indicated no significant relationships between demographic variables and ADL abilities at admission or at discharge. Length of stay was significantly related to ADL abilities upon admission ($r = -.36$, $p<.05$) and at discharge ($r = -.22$, $p<.05$), such that longer lengths of stay were associated with decreased ADL abilities. The number of chronic medical conditions was also significantly related to ADL abilities upon admission ($r = -.14$, $p<.05$) and at discharge ($r = -.15$, $p<.05$), such that having more medical conditions was related to decreased ADL abilities. Finally, cognition was significantly related to ADL abilities upon admission ($r = .22$, $p<.05$), and at discharge ($r = .30$, $p<.05$).

In Table 2.1 the results for the prediction of discharge ADL abilities are presented. Variables were entered in four blocks for this hierarchical regression analysis. ADL scores at admission were entered first, demographic variables second (age, race, education, and gender), and number of existing medical conditions and length of stay were entered third. Cognition was entered last. Admission ADLs accounted for 53 percent of the variance in discharge ADL skills. Variables in steps 2 and 3 did not significantly add to the prediction of discharge ADL scores. Cognition, however, significantly added 3 percent of variance. Results of this study confirmed that cognition is related to physical recovery during medical rehabilitation. In order to test the stability of these conclusions, a third study was conducted in this area. In this study, Charlene Moore (1994), for her dissertation thesis, explored the data through regression analysis and executed a cross validation and double cross-validation procedure.

TABLE 2.1. Stepwise Hierarchical Regressions of Demographic, Medical, Cognitive, and Affective Measures on Discharge Activities of Daily Living (ADL) Skills

Step	Variable	Beta	t	Sig. t	R^2 Change	Cumulative R^2
1.	Admission ADL	−.73	282.78	.00	.53***	.53***
2.	Race[a]	−.00	−.00	.96	—	—
	Sex[b]	−.10	5.69	.02	—	—
	Age	.04	.74	.39	—	—
	Education	.07	2.27	.14	—	—
	Block	—	—	—	.01	.54***
3.	Number of Medical Conds.	.03	.54	.46	—	—
	LOS	−.06	1.85	.18	—	—
	Block	—	—	—	.00	.55***
4.	DRS	.19	16.25	.00	.03*	.58***

Note: [a]   Race was dummy coded 0 = black and 1 = white.
          [b]   Sex was dummy coded 0 = male and 1 = female.
          * $p < .05$
          *** $p < .001$

The sample for this study consisted of 154 geriatric medical rehabilitation inpatients (Moore and Lichtenberg, 1995). Forty-six subjects were male and 108 female, with 86 African Americans and 56 Caucasians; data were missing on race for 12 of the subjects. Mean age was 77.33 (SD = 7.19; range 62–95). Average educational level was 10.12 (SD = 3.29; range 0–20). In this study data were collected on a number of neuropsychological tests, in addition to the Mattis Dementia Rating Scale. Preliminary analyses, however, revealed strong correlations (e.g., most were greater than .70) between the neuropsychological variables. To counteract multicollinearity, forming a composite score (labeled NCOMP) was chosen because it improves the reliability of the results. It also allows for a fuller representation of the domain of interest, cognitive functioning. Thus the variable chosen treats cognition as a global variable.

For the purposes of cross validation of regression results, the data set was randomly divided into two equal groups of 77 subjects each. Analyses of the two groups for differences in mean values for age, education, Boston Naming Test, Dementia Rating Scale, Logical Memory I and II, Index of Comorbidity, and FIM score were performed through the use of T-tests. In addition, possible differences in representation of gender and ethnic heritage were analyzed through X^2 tests. No significant differences between groups were noted for any of the variables analyzed.

A multiple regression analysis predicting FIM scores was conducted. Using a hierarchical entry method, demographic variables (i.e., age, education, and gender) for the first group of subjects were entered into the equation. The R^2 value, representing the total proportion of the variance accounted for by the model, was 0.12 following this entry. The Index of Comorbidity (CMI) (Charlson, 1987) was then entered into the equation, resulting in no significant change in R^2. On the final step, NCOMP was entered, increasing the amount of variance accounted for to 18 percent—an additional 6 percent. Final standardized beta weights, standard errors, and associated F-tests for these equations by group are presented in Table 2.2. The strongest noted beta weight in this equation was that for the neuropsychological composite score, at .32, with that of education next highest at -0.27. F values on all entered variables indicated that only these two variables were significant predictors of FIM scores for this group.

The entry method above was also used for the second group of subjects (n = 77). Following entry of demographic variables for this group, R^2 was 0.01. Entry of CMI increased this to 0.25. On the final step, NCOMP increased the R^2 an additional 3 percent to 0.28.

Double Cross Validation of Regression Equations

In order to determine the stability of the observed regression weights in the two equations described above, a double cross validation study was undertaken. In this procedure, predicted FIM scores for each group were obtained by entering the B weights and constant value achieved from the equation for the other group. Pearson correlations between the resulting predicted scores and observed FIM scores were then calculated and compared to the multiple R for each equation. The application of equation 1 to group 1 revealed no shrinkage, with the correlation between observed FIM scores and predicted scores equal to 0.536. This result was comparable to a final multiple R for group 2 of .53598. The equation developed based on group 1, however, revealed a decrease

TABLE 2.2. Final Results of Multiple Regression Analysis by Group

	B Wt.	SE B	Beta	T	Sign.T
Group 1:					
Gender	3.64	2.62	.1515	1.39	.17
Education	−0.86	0.36	−.2717	−2.35	.02
Age	−0.19	0.22	−.1109	−0.86	.39
CMI	0.21	1.65	.0141	0.13	.90
NCOMP	0.70	0.29	.3218	2.38	.02
(CONSTANT)	75.58	18.70		4.04	.01
Group 2:					
Gender	0.79	2.34	.0348	−.34	.74
Education	−0.54	0.38	−.1581	−1.43	.16
Age	0.03	0.14	.0240	.22	.83
CMI	−6.32	1.34	−.4855	−4.70	.01
NCOMP	0.38	0.20	.2145	1.90	.06
(CONSTANT)	66.22	12.94		5.11	.01
Full Data Set:					
Gender	2.30	1.78	−.0985	1.29	.20
Education	−0.82	.27	−.2504	−3.08	.01
Age	−0.05	.13	.0356	−0.42	.68
CMI	−3.11	1.08	−.2246	−2.88	.01
NCOMP	.55	.17	.2811	3.18	.01
(CONSTANT)	69.57	11.09		6.27	.01

Note: CMI   = Comorbidity Index
NCOMP = Neuropsychological Composite Score

in the amount of variance accounted for; the initial equation accounted for 18.1 percent of the variance. When applied to group 2, variance accounted for was reduced to only 2.4 percent.

Multiple Regression on Full Data Set

Using an entry method identical to that described above, a multiple regression was then performed on data for all subjects. Following entry of demographic variables, R^2 was 0.03. Entry of CMI followed, with an increase in R^2 to 0.09. Finally, entry of NCOMP increased R^2 to 0.15. Observed beta weights ranged from −0.2246 to 0.2811. T-tests on all entered variables indicated that education

(T_{153} = –3.08, p = .0025), CMI (T_{153} = –2.881; p = .0046), and NCOMP (T_{153} = 3.182; p = .0018) were all significant predictors of FIM score for the full sample. For the full data set, the regression equation was FIM = 69.57 + (2.3)Gender + (–.82)Education + (–.05)Age + (–3.11)CMI + (.55)NCOMP.

The equation derived from group 1 showed a significant amount of shrinkage when applied to group 2, indicating an instability of the B weights derived from group 1. However, the equation derived from group 2 showed no shrinkage, indicating good stability of the derived equation. The most significant predictor from this equation was the Comorbidity Index; this index also proved to be highly significant when predicting scores for the entire data set. Neuro-psychological variables also proved to be significant predictors of ADL performance. There was, however, a great deal of variability in this score; the standard deviation was greater than or equal to the mean. It appears, however, that information about a patient's medical history and current medical diagnoses can be powerful indicators of a patient's ability to attend to his or her own self-care. These results underscore the need for routinely obtaining this information about patients for whom input is requested regarding their ability to live independently.

CLINICAL IMPLICATIONS OF REHABILITATION AND ADL STUDIES

Older medical rehabilitation patients, too often, have only their mechanical functioning assessed (e.g., gait, balance, strength, range of motion) in determining their potential physical progress, as well as their potential for independent living and autonomy. The results of our studies indicated that cognitive aspects of functioning are also important to address. Utilizing new techniques for grooming, bathing, transferring from bed to chair, etc., all require the interaction of planning, visuomotor, attentional, and memory skills. It is not surprising then that cognition emerged as a strong predictor of these skills, particularly in the impaired patients. Cognition, as an indirect measure of brain functioning and a direct measure of mental performance, should be an integral part of the multidiscipinary assessment in health care settings. Depending on the interaction

between cognitive performance and the physical ability requirements in a patient's environment, appropriate treatment goals can
be set. Too often, patient goals are set unrealistically high for a
demented patient whose physical disabilities are relatively straightforward, but whose cognition was never assessed and whose
dementia never realized. In these cases, the patients lack the necessary cognitive skills to perform multistep behaviors such as dressing, grooming, or transferring.

THE RELATIONSHIP OF NEUROPSYCHOLOGICAL VARIABLES TO INSTRUMENTAL ACTIVITIES OF DAILY LIVING SKILLS (IADLS)

Instrumental activities are construed as those more advanced
ADL tasks that are necessary for independent living (Lawton and
Brody, 1969). These typically include using the telephone, shopping, meal preparation, cleaning, laundry, use of transportation,
handling finances, and medication adherence. The importance of
these skills was underscored by the finding that poor performance
on advanced daily living tasks was one of the strongest predictors of
nursing home placement in an epidemiological study of 3,646 older
adults (Wolinsky et al., 1993). Recent research has explored the
relationship of cognitive variables with IADL abilities.

Palmer and Dobson (1994) investigated the relationship between
memory functioning and accuracy in self-medication in a geriatric
medical rehabilitation program. Specifically, two stages were investigated: the ability of patients to ask nurses for their medication,
and, if successful in stage 1, the ability to comply with a 24-hour
supply of medication. A discriminant function analysis was able to
correctly identify 95 percent of those patients who completed both
stages (i.e., independent with medication), and 100 percent of those
unable to complete stage 1 (i.e., not independent with medication).
Sixty-four percent of the variance was accounted for by three cognitive tests: block design, short delayed recall on the California Verbal
Learning Test, and self-rated memory ability. Isaac and Tamblyn
(1993) also reported similar findings to the above study when they
investigated visuospatial problem-solving tasks, a memory task,
and accurate medication compliance in 20 outpatients.

Performance-based driving skills were investigated in 24 normal and 6 demented drivers having a mean age of 72 years (Odenheimer et al., 1994). Interrater reliability of subjects driving ability was .84 on the 10-mile, 45-minute road test. Driving was rated as unsafe, safe in optimal conditions only, or safe. The Mini Mental State Exam (MMSE) was significantly related to the driving score (r = .72, p<.05), as was memory functioning (r = .51, p<.05) and complex reaction time (r = .70, p<.05). All of the demented drivers displayed unsafe driving skills. An alternative method of studying driving ability is by utilizing motor vehicle accident frequency as the criterion variable (Owsley et al., 1991).

These researchers were investigating why there was such a poor link between visual acuity and driving accidents. A total of 53 participants, all primary care patients at an optometry school, were included in the study. The participants had a mean age of 70 years and drove at least 1,000 miles per year. Visual abilities were measured across several factors including acuity, contrast sensitivity, and field of view. In addition, a mental status test—the Mattis Organic Mental Status Syndrome Examination—was obtained (Mattis 1976). On each mental status exam subtest, subjects were scored on a scale ranging from impaired to normal. Driving data were obtained from the state department of public safety. Significant correlations were found between useful field of view and accident frequency (r = .36, p<.05) and mental status and accident frequency (r = .34, p<.05). Better field of view and better mental status scores were related to fewer accidents. Mental status and useful field of view were significantly related to one another as well (r = .32, p<.05). Taken together, these two variables accounted for 20 percent of accident frequency variance in a regression equation.

Several recent studies have documented the significant relationship between cognition and IADLs in samples of white older adults. In studies described more fully in the ADL section of Nadler et al.'s 1991 work, Nadler and colleagues found the Dementia Rating Scale to be significantly related to money management (r = .52, p<.05) and to medication administration (r = .64, p<.05). In their follow-up study, this pattern of results held (Richardson, Nadler, and Molloy, 1995). The Hooper visual organization test (VOT), for example, was significantly related to safety (r = .50, p<.05), medication administration (r = .61, p<.05), cooking (r = .28, p<.05), and money management (r = .39, p<.05). This pattern of relationships between cognitive measures and IADL abilities held for other tests, such as Logical Memory and Visual Reproduction logical memory subtests from the Wechsler Memory Scale–Revised. In a similar study, Loewenstein et al. (1992) reported that the Mini Mental State Exam was significantly correlated with phone usage (r = .46, p<.05), counting money (r = .62, p<.05), and using the checkbook (r = .43, p<.05).

Although the results of the above investigations report converging data on the relationship of cognition to IADL abilities, there are limitations to these data. Much of the data has been collected on psychogeriatric patients or community volunteers. The findings cannot, thus, be generalized to older adult medical samples. In addition, there was a lack of urban medical subjects in these samples, and thus the generalizability of the above results is limited. Finally, there has been little conceptual progress in the past five years regarding the relationship between IADLs and cognition. No study has proposed new variables that might add to the prediction of IADL skills. A former colleague at the University of Virginia, Tony Giuliano, hypothesized that by measuring awareness of deficit, we could improve the prediction of IADLs and advance clinical practice because, he reasoned, without awareness, there would be no compensation for deficits, thereby leading to mistakes. Jennifer Caron (1996) studied these variables in her dissertation thesis.

Awareness of Deficit

Babinski (1914) used the term "anosognosia" to describe the failure to recognize a disease state. Two of his patients denied paralysis of their arm despite good cognitive functioning. Heilman (1991) postulated that anosognosia is caused by a failure in self-monitoring, which is believed to be largely controlled by the frontal cortex. It has only been in the last 15 years that awareness of deficit has been more thoroughly described and studied in cases of progressive dementia.

A loss of insight, or lacking awareness of cognitive deficits, has been described in the middle and later stages of cortical dementias (Bergmann, Proctor, and Prudham, 1979; Reisberg et al., 1985). During the middle phase of Alzheimer's disease, the confusional phase, initial loss of insight regarding memory difficulties was noted by Reisberg and his colleagues. Other researchers reported converging data—that as the dementia progressed, the lack of insight increased (Gustafson and Nilsson, 1982; Mangone et al., 1991).

Other research, however, has suggested that lack of awareness of deficit can come early in a dementing process. Green, Goldstein, Sirockman, and Green (1991) reported that early dementia patients reported having far greater abilities as compared to their family member's report. Still, other studies suggest that with vascular dementia or subcortical dementia, for example, insight into deficits is retained (Danielczyk, 1983; DeBettignies, Mahurin, and Pirozzolo, 1990). Several methodological limitations of these studies were evident. Many studies failed to include objective measures of performance when examining awareness, relying instead on patient and family report. There were measurement shortcomings in the above studies. The most critical issues were the usage of subjective ratings by the examiner without ensuring interrater reliability or using a psychometrically sound instrument. Degree of cognitive impairment was not controlled for, and the predictive abilities of awareness of deficit were not studied. Caron and Lichtenberg (1996) remediated several of these problems by investigating the relationship between awareness of deficit, cognitive functioning, and subjective and objective IADL skills in urban older adult medical patients.

Study to Predict IADLs

Measures used for the awareness of deficit variable and for the IADL variable will be described first. The sample and results will then be discussed. Patients' subjective perceptions of their cognitive and neuropsychological performance was assessed by the Awareness Interview (Anderson and Tranel, 1989). The Awareness Interview is composed of two parts. The first part is administered orally to patients before they have undertaken any cognitive or IADL tasks. We utilized six items that were scored on a three-point scale (1 through 3). These items assess the patient's beliefs about his or her abilities in the following areas: reason for hospitalization, general cognitive functioning, orientation, memory, speech and language abilities, and visual perception. The second part of the interview is administered orally to the patient after he or she has completed cognitive testing. It consists of one category: a self-evaluation of the patient's performance on the cognitive testing.

Scoring of the Awareness Interview depends upon a combination of the self-ratings described above and the objective test data supplied by the cognitive testing. Test data corresponding to each of the six domains of functioning assessed by the Awareness Interview can be obtained by using the Normative Studies Research Project (NSRP) test battery. Impairment on neuropsychological measures was determined according to the number of standard deviations from established norms (see NSRP test battery for normative data). Scores within one standard deviation of the mean were considered unimpaired. Scores within one to two standard deviations from the mean were considered mildly impaired, and scores greater than two standard deviations from the mean were considered maximally impaired.

Deviation scores were calculated by subtracting Awareness Interview self-ratings from objective neuropsychological test ratings. The deviation scores were then added together to form an Awareness Index with values ranging from 0 through 14. An Awareness Index of 0 means that the patient has no cognitive deficits, or that they were able to accurately describe their cognitive impairments. A score of 14 was interpreted as revealing severe unawareness of deficit (i.e., no agreement between subjective ratings and objective test scores).

Patients' ability to perform their IADLs was assessed by a revised form of the Structured Assessment of Independent Living Skills (SAILS) (Mahurin, DeBettignies, and Priozzolo, 1991). The IADL components of the SAILS utilized in this study included money management, telephone use, medication management, and basic cooking. A total IADL index was calculated by summing scores on the subscales for each patient, with a range of possible scores ranging from 0 to 30.

The SAILS was chosen for this study particularly because it was designed to assess IADL functioning in persons suspected of having a dementia, and for its good reliability and validity data (Mahurin, DeBettignies, and Priozzolo, 1991). Test retest reliability for normal elderly and for those with Alzheimer's disease was $r = .81$ and $r = .99$ respectively. Internal consistency of the scale was also excellent (r = .90, p<.05). Using discriminant function analysis, the SAILS money-related skill items were significantly different between normal patients and Alzheimer's patients. Finally, concurrent validity with the Full Scale IQ on the Wechsler Adult Intelligence Scale–Revised was high (r = .79, p<.05).

Fifty older adult medical rehabilitation patients formed the sample for this investigation. The mean age was 78 years (SD = 8.5), and mean education was 10 years (SD = 3.4). Sixty-four percent of the patients were women and 36 percent were men; and 68 percent of the patients were African American and 32 percent were white. Results of correlational analyses among variables can be found in Table 2.3. As can be seen in the table, cognition held the strongest relationship to performance on the SAILS (r = .75, p<.05), followed by awareness of deficit (r = .69, p<.05), and education (r = .57, p<.05). Age, race, and sex were unrelated to SAILS scores. In addition, self-reported IADL abilities were unrelated to SAILS scores. Cognition was highly related to awareness of deficit (r = –.72, p<.05) such that the more cognitive problems an individual had the more unrealistic they were in appraising their abilities.

Regression analyses were used to test the predictive abilities of neuropsychological and awareness-of-deficit variables (in measuring performance-based IADLs) once self-reported IADLs and demographic abilities were accounted for. Blocks were entered into a hierarchical regression in the prediction of SAILS scores (see Table 2.4). In the first block, self-reported IADL scores were entered. This variable was not a significant predictor of SAILS scores. In the second block, the demographic variables of age, gender, race, and education were entered. Education was a significant predictor of SAILS scores, and together the block accounted for 29 percent of SAILS variance. In the third block, cognition was entered. The DRS was a significant predictor of SAILS scores and accounted for 28 percent of unique SAILS variance above and beyond the effects of self-reported IADL and demographic predictors. The awareness-of-deficit score was entered in the final block of the regression so as to examine whether it provided any unique prediction of SAILS scores. Awareness of deficit was a significant predictor of SAILS scores, accounting for 7 percent of SAILS variance above and beyond that accounted for by all the other predictors.

TABLE 2.3. Correlations

	Age	AI	DRS	Education	Sex	IADL	Race	SAILS
Age	—							
AI	-.02	—						
DRS	-.14	-.72***	—					
Education	-.25#	-.28*	.47***	—				
Sex[a]	-.01	-.02	.08	.17	—			
IADL	-.06	-.09	.08	.32*	.13	—		
Race[b]	.26#	.23	-.29*	-.21	.18	-.18	—	
SAILS	-.22	-.69***	.75***	.57***	.17	.32*	-.31*	—

Note: a Sex was coded ___ male, ___ female.
b Race was coded 1 = African American, 2 = white.
# p < .10
* p < .05
*** p < .001

TABLE 2.4. Stepwise Hierarchical Regressions of Measures on SAILS

Step	Variable	Beta	t	Sig. t	R^2 Change	Cumulative R^2
1.	IADL	.25	1.82	.08	.06#	.06#
2.	Race[a]	−.20	−1.54	.13	—	—
	Sex[b]	.10	.78	.44	—	—
	Age	−.03	−.27	.79	—	—
	Education	.46	3.46	.001	—	—
	Block	—	—	—	.29**	.35***
3.	DRS	.63	5.81	.001	.29***	.64***
4.	AI	−.36	−2.91	.01	.06**	.70***

Notes: [a] Race was dummy coded ( ) = black, ( ) = white.
      [b] Sex was dummy coded ( ) = male, ( ) = female.
      ** $p < .05$
      *** $p < .001$

While this study produced exciting results that the clinician can use, there were some limitations. Sample size was the chief limitation. The sample is small, and the relationships found here must be validated on larger samples. With larger samples, for example, it is likely that the magnitude of the correlations will be reduced, and that the regression analysis will not account for as much of the variance. Nevertheless, this study added two new main findings to our knowledge about the ecological validity of neuropsychological variables in an older urban medical population: Cognitive tests are significant predictors of IADL abilities, and awareness of deficit, although highly related to cognition, provides additional prediction of IADL abilities.

Evaluating the ability to return to independent living, particularly in those that live alone, is a frequent referral task in health care settings. Despite its importance, we found only one published study that investigated the cognitive factors associated with return to living alone. Friedman (1993) prospectively studied 178 older adults who were living alone and had a stroke. The surviving patients were followed at 2, 6, and 12 months poststroke. Thirty-three percent of patients were discharged back to living alone, and this number remained constant throughout the 12-month follow-up period. In comparing those who returned to living alone versus those who did not, ADL abilities, MMSE score, and type of stroke (lacunar versus nonlacunar) were the most powerful predictors. This study was conducted in New Zealand, however, and thus has limited generalizability in the United States since health care systems may be dramatically different between the two countries.

My colleague, Susan MacNeill, and I conducted a study in order to better assess the relationship between cognition, ADL abilities, and return to living alone in an older adult medical rehabilitation sample (MacNeill and Lichtenberg, in press). Three hundred seventy-two patients who entered the hospital and were living alone prior to admission were studied. Similar to our other studies, this group had a mean age of 78 years (SD = 7.9), consisted of 75 percent women, and two-thirds were African American.

One hundred forty-six (39 percent) of patients returned to live alone after their hospitalization. Logistic regression with a forward-selection forced-entry method was utilized to determine what were the best predictors of return to living alone. When ADL and ambulation abilities were entered first, there was a 63 percent overall correct rate of classification. Demographic variables and co-morbid medical disease were entered on the next two steps, but did not improve prediction. Finally, the DRS total score was entered. Classification improved by 9 percent overall to 72 percent. The Chi Square values for the different predictors can be found in Table 2.5.

In order to further test the ability of DRS scores to predict return to living alone, three ranges of scores were examined. The severely impaired group (DRS<101), the moderate to mildly impaired group (101<DRS<125), and the unimpaired group (DRS>125). Only 20 percent of the severely impaired group returned to live alone, and only 30 percent of the moderate to mildly impaired group returned to live alone. In contrast, 52 percent of the unimpaired group returned to living alone. Further analysis revealed that ADL abilities were unrelated to discharge status in the severely impaired group, but were related to discharge status in the other two groups. We concluded that cognition is the vital limiting factor in preventing older adults with severe cognitive limitations from returning to living alone. An interaction between cognition and functioning is present in the other group.

TABLE 2.5. Predictors of Discharge Disposition (Home Alone Compared to Those Not Discharged Home Alone)

Variable	Chi-Square	p
FIM Admission Score	37.544	.0000
DRS Total Score	16.702	.0000
Demographic Variables	9.240	.0554
Medical Burden	.013	.9104

Note: Variables are ranked according to chi-square values.

CLINICAL IMPLICATIONS OF IADL RESEARCH

Quite often mental health practitioners are questioned as to the applicability of their test findings to real-world behaviors. "Well he was living alone before," or "Yes, but in his own environment he could manage himself" are frequent challenges to the usage of cognitive assessment data in treatment planning. The IADL literature reviewed and the studies conducted by our research group, in particular, can be used to offset these arguments. The validity of applying cognitive assessment results, along with other relevant medical, biographical, and social information is supported. In the areas of driving and medication compliance, the role of cognition is clear. In those patients who were demented and had documented memory disturbance, driving performance and medication compliance was substandard.

The IADL and living alone studies were perhaps the most unique. In the Caron and Lichtenberg study, a direct relationship was found between cognition and IADL abilities. What was even more useful, however, was that awareness of deficit emerged as a variable with clinical significance and utility. How aware a patient was of any cognitive deficits was related to their IADL performance. This makes sense since without awareness there is no compensation. Those individuals who had cognitive deficits but were aware of these shortcomings were able to compensate, at least partially, for the cognitive deficits, and to perform the IADLs. Awareness of deficit should emerge as a routine aspect of the clinical evaluation.

MacNeill and Lichtenberg (in press) performed a truly unique study aimed at identifying the aspects of a patient's condition that led them to return home alone. The most useful predictor of whether a patient was able to go home alone or not was cognition. That is, even in an environment that was focused on basic ADLs and locomotion, cognition was still the most critical variable in discharge outcome. The assessment of cognitive functioning ought to become an integral part of discharge planning in health care settings.

SUMMARY

We reviewed the research of others, as well as our own data that indicate the central role of cognition in determining physical recovery of ADL skills, in predicting the ability to engage in advanced self-care tasks and in forecasting discharge status in those that live alone. Cognition, thus, is a central variable in functional and living status of older adults.

We introduced new topics into research that can be of value to clinicians. The measurement and usage of awareness of deficit in predicting self-care tasks adds unique information to assessing only cognition. Clinicians are well advised to begin utilizing this construct and measuring it in their clinical work. The central role of cognition in predicting ability to return to living alone is a unique contribution to the gerontology literature. These data set the stage for more research on ecological validity of neuropsychological tests in older adults.

Chapter 3

The Role of Depression
in Geriatric Health Outcomes

Depression is a health concern, not just a mental health concern. This chapter will review the literature on the links between depression and medical burden, and the links between depression and physical health in older adults. Studies conducted on our urban samples will be described, methods of measuring depression will be discussed, and the empirical results of our behavioral treatment program will be analyzed. The significance of depression in the context of health care settings will be amplified, both by its prevalence and its effects on health outcomes. In this chapter, the empirical evidence to support the link between depression and health outcomes is presented, and in a later chapter, the specific method of depression treatment will be described.

PREVALENCE OF DEPRESSION
IN MEDICALLY ILL OLDER ADULTS

Depression in the physically ill elder is a common problem. Two large epidemiological studies of community elderly revealed that major depression is rare in community elders compared with medically ill and institutionalized elderly (Blazer, Hughes, and George, 1987; Kramer et al., 1985). In a survey of over 3,000 cases, the Kramer group reported 0.7 percent of those age 65 to 74 suffered from major depression and 1.3 percent of those age 75 and over suffered from major depression. Blazer, Hughes, and George (1987) reported very similar results with regard to major depressive illness.

Blazer and his colleagues did find the rate for dysphoria, however, to be 19 percent.

In light of these findings in the community elderly, it is significant to find that 20 years of research has consistently documented elderly medical outpatients and inpatients to have depression rates ranging from 15 to 45 percent (Kitchell et al., 1982; Norris et al., 1987; Okimoto et al., 1982; Rapp, Parisi, and Walsh, 1988; Schuckit, Miller, and Hahlbohn, 1975; Waxman and Carner, 1984), making it at least significantly more prevalent in this group.

Several points must be kept in mind when interpreting these studies, however. All but one of the studies was conducted on a male veteran population, and only two studies included a sizeable sample of women. Second, it was only in the Rapp et al. (1988) study that the reliability and validity of the diagnostic interview results were assessed.

Our research has focused on depression in medical rehabilitation patients. Lichtenberg et al. (1993) investigated the prevalence of depression in 150 geriatric medical rehabilitation inpatients, utilizing the Geriatric Depression Scale and a clinical interview for Research Diagnostic Criteria (Spitzer and Endicott, 1979). The overall prevalence rate for major and minor depression was 34 percent. In a follow-up study, Hanks and Lichtenberg (1996) utilized 812 geriatric medical rehabilitation inpatients and found a 30 percent prevalence for depression.

Depression in medically ill patients has consistently been under-recognized by primary physicians, particularly with the elderly medical patient. This finding of poor detection of mental health problems in older medical patients is applicable to cognitive disorders and substance abuse disorders. In a sample of 96 family medicine outpatients, physicians accurately detected only 22 percent of existing depression (Moore, Silimperi, and Bobula, 1978). Nielsen and Williams (1980) reported that in a sample of 526 outpatients only 10 percent were correctly diagnosed with depression by their physicians. Waxman and Carner (1984) and Rapp et al. (1988) reported on samples of only elderly medically ill patients with comparable findings. In the Waxman and Carner study, physicians correctly identified only 11 percent of those who were depressed. In the Rapp study only 8.7 percent of depressed patients were correctly identified by the primary physician. In regard to medical rehabilitation inpatients, Lichtenberg et al. (1993) found that physicians detected depression in 50 percent of depressed female patients, and detected depression in only 10 percent of depressed male patients. In conclusion, depression is a prevalent but poorly understood problem in geriatric rehabilitation. In the sections that follow, it will become clear that although depression is often ignored by health care professionals, it is a primary predictor of functional status and functional recovery, consistent with the discussion of cognition in the previous chapter. Thus, depression is a health problem that needs to be treated effectively.

MEASURING DEPRESSION IN URBAN ELDERLY: THE GERIATRIC DEPRESSION SCALE

The Geriatric Depression Scale (GDS) was created in the early 1980s (Brink et al., 1982; Yesavage et al., 1983) and was the first screening measure developed for and validated on the elderly. The GDS is composed of 30 yes/no self-referent statements. An advantage of the GDS over other self-report measures is its omission (on an empirical basis) of somatic items. The GDS has been found to be a highly reliable and valid measure of depression in the elderly. Acceptable levels of reliability have been reported by Brink and his colleagues, and by Rapp, Parisi, Walsh, and Wallace (1988). This scale has also been demonstrated to be useful in detecting depression in medically ill elderly with improved sensitivity/specificity data compared to other self-report measures (Norris et al., 1987; Rapp, Parisi, and Walsh, 1988). There is also considerable evidence that the GDS is valid when used with cognitively compromised patients (Parmelee, Katz, and Lawton, 1989; Lichtenberg et al., 1992), although these findings are not unequivocal (Kafonek et al., 1989).

The utility of the Geriatric Depression Scale in urban elderly was assessed in a sample of 313 patients. Reliability and validity of the GDS were measured through Chronbach's alpha (internal consistency) and through factor analysis. Internal consistency was found to be extremely good (alpha = .86), meaning that individual items correlated well with the total score. Thus the items on the GDS were interpreted as measuring the same construct. Factor analysis of the GDS revealed nine factors. Although this was three more factors than were uncovered in previous research, the main factors identified by us were the same as identified in previous research: life dissatisfaction and hopelessness.

THE RELATIONSHIP OF DEPRESSION
TO PHYSICAL HEALTH OUTCOMES

Livingston Bruce et al. (1994) used community-based cohorts from the National Institute on Aging's Established Populations for Epidemiological Studies of the Elderly (EPESE) to follow 1,189 older adults. The cohort was interviewed in 1988 and again approximately 2.5 years later. Subject mortality from refusals and deaths was 6 percent (n = 73). Initially, all subjects were independent in all activities of daily living. At the second interview, 5.7 percent men and 4.1 percent women had disabilities with regards to activities of daily living. For both men and women, when controlling for other medical factors, depression emerged as a significant predictor of disability onset.

Depression appears to be a significant factor in long-term recovery among geriatric stroke patients. Depression may be twice as common in poststroke patients as it is in community elderly (Primeau, 1988). Parikh et al. (1990) studied the relationship of depression to ADL functioning two years following the initial stroke. Patients who had been depressed in the hospital were significantly more impaired in physical activities two years after their stroke than were the nondepressed patients. Bacher et al. (1990) reported similar findings in their 12-month study of 48 poststroke patients. None of the above studies, however, controlled for demographic influences on recovery, nor investigated the role of rehabilitation in recovery.

Other researchers have demonstrated a relationship between functional recovery and depression in geriatric patients following orthopedic injuries. Reduced recovery from hip fracture was associated with depression in a number of studies. Among these, Cummings et al. (1988) provided a six-month follow-up of 92 hip fracture patients. Depressive symptomatology was associated with poorer outcome in basic and advanced activities of daily living one year after hip fracture in a sample of 536 geriatric patients assessed by Magaziner et al. (1990).

Diamond et al. (1995) investigated the effects of depression on functional outcome during geriatric physical rehabilitation. Depression was prevalent in 29.4 percent of the sample at admission, and in 22 percent of the sample at discharge from a 25-day rehabilitation stay. While the depressed and nondepressed patients did not differ on functional abilities at admission, the depressed patients made fewer gains at discharge. It is important to note here that without any treatment during their rehabilitation, patients by and large remained depressed.

Methodological weaknesses of the above studies were numerous. Most importantly, these studies failed to control for potential moderator variables such as age, education, sex, and the severity of patients' medical problems. With the exception of the Diamond study, none of the studies investigated the role of rehabilitation in the depression-functional recovery relationship. Our research has focused on this issue utilizing two samples: a preliminary study of 52 patients, and a follow-up study of 423 patients. The characteristics of the sample with 423 patients was the same one described in the previous chapter on cognition.

The studies to be presented here provide evidence that depression among elderly is an important risk factor for failure to recover following illness or injury. We conducted two studies to determine whether depression was a relevant variable in physical recovery, with emphasis on the potential role of depression in activities of daily living skills at the end of rehabilitation (Lichtenberg et al., 1994). In the first study, 52 participants were utilized. A series of hierarchical regression analyses were used to determine whether depression was a unique and significant predictor of activities of daily living on admission to and discharge from an inpatient rehabilitation program. In the first block of the regression analysis, demographic variables were entered. The second block of predictors included length of stay and the number of comorbid medical conditions. The third predictor block consisted of a cognitive functioning measure. Finally, depression was entered in the fourth block of the analysis. The results indicated that whereas depression was not a significant predictor of activities of daily living upon admission to rehabilitation, depression was a predictor of discharge activities of daily living. Thus, levels of depression were a significant predictor of functional recovery during rehabilitation.

Nanna et al. (in press) improved upon the above study's methodology by increasing the sample size to 423 participants and by controlling for initial level of activities of daily living functioning. On the first step of the regression analysis, admission activities of daily living ability were entered. This was followed by blocks of demographic data, medical data, and cognitive data. Finally, depression was entered on the last step of the regression equation. The findings of this study replicated the earlier results and led to the conclusion that depression is a key variable that helps to determine physical functioning outcomes during the rehabilitation process.

The effects of depression on survival in our geriatric medical rehabilitation population was assessed by examining survival to 1996 for those patients admitted between 1991 and 1993. Four hundred fifty-five subjects, representing consecutive admissions to the geriatric rehabilitation program, who received both a cognitive assessment (i.e., the Dementia Rating Scale) and an affective assessment (i.e., the Geriatric Depression Scale), were entered into the survival analysis. The study examined univariate and multivariate predictors of survival. The yearly mortality rate was 19 percent, with an overall mortality rate of 36 percent. Predictor variables included demographic variables, medical burden, ADL abilities, length of stay, and Dementia Rating Scale and Geriatric Depression Scale scores. Univariate analyses found that two variables demonstrated a higher relative risk for death (depression score and medical burden), whereas three variables produced protective effects against death: being female, increased ADL abilities, and higher Dementia Rating Scale scores. In the multivariate analysis, however, only two variables predicted survival: depression score and sex. Depression was the best predictor of survival when compared to all other predictor variables. The relative risk of dying was 38 percent higher for those with higher depression scores as opposed to those with lower scores.

The general conclusion drawn from these studies was that depression is a significant predictor of important health outcomes: activities of daily living and mortality. A logical next step was to attempt to treat depression and thereby improve both mood and health outcomes.

PSYCHOSOCIAL TREATMENT
OF GERIATRIC DEPRESSION

Scogin and McElreath (1994) summarized many of the previous studies of depression treatment with older adults by performing a meta-analysis of published empirical studies. A total of 17 studies were included in their analysis, and each of these studies compared a treatment group to a no-treatment control group. Mean age for the subjects was 70.5 years and there was a mean education of 12.6 years. Mean effect size was 1.22, indicative of moderate to good success in depression treatment. These data were consistent with other meta-analytic studies conducted on younger depressed patients. The authors concluded that psychosocial interventions for older adults experiencing depressive symptoms are effective.

Rattenbury and Stones (1989) compared two reminiscence treatment groups (based on Butler's Life Review theories) to a no-treatment control group in a sample with a mean age above 83 years. This is one of the few studies reported that focused on depression in the oldest adults in our society. The researchers reported that the data provided support for the intervention, specifically that patients' levels of depression were reduced and their mood improved. There were no global improvements in physical functioning, however.

While the results of the studies reviewed by Scogin and McElreath (1994) provide support for psychological therapies with depression, there are shortcomings to these data. While most studies used blind raters and random assignment to groups, none of the treatment studies reviewed by Scogin and McElreath targeted geriatric medical patients suffering from depression. The vast majority of the studies had a mean subject age in the sixties (and only one over age 80). None of the treatments included patients from minority groups. Thus, generalizability of the above findings to medical rehabilitation inpatients, to an African-American sample, and to the oldest old is questionable.

The behavioral theory of depression was chosen as the one to guide treatment research with older urban medical patients. This approach was chosen for several reasons. First, there is a 25-year history of empirical support for this theory. Second, the theory has been applied successfully to older adults. Third, the behavioral approach focuses upon identifying clear goals and specific activities for patients to engage in. Finally, its focus on daily events translates well to a medical setting, and is easy to explain to other interdisciplinary team members.

BEHAVIORAL THEORY OF DEPRESSION

The Behavioral Theory of Depression, as described by Lewinsohn and his colleagues, offers a rationale for depression treatment that is supported by a series of empirical studies. The theory characterizes the maintenance of depression as "a series of person-environment interactions characterized by a deficit in positive experiences and an excess of aversive ones" (Teri and Gallagher-Thompson, 1991, p. 414). Basically, then, depression is maintained by an excess of unpleasant events and a lack of pleasant ones.

During the past 20 years, Lewinsohn and colleagues have provided empirical support for their theory. Lewinsohn and Graf (1973) presented preliminary data that for young, middle-aged, and older adults, pleasant events were significantly related to mood. Lewinsohn and Talkington (1979) created a 160-item pleasant events schedule that demonstrated reliability and validity. Teri and Lewinsohn (1982) then adapted this scale to the elderly, and later, Teri and Logsdon (1991) adapted the scale for dementia patients. In all of the studies mentioned here, pleasant activities were significantly related to depression measures such that the greater the number of pleasant events the lower the depression.

Thompson, Gallagher, and Breckenridge (1987) compared the effectiveness of behavioral treatment with cognitive and psychodynamic treatment for depression in older adults. Each treatment group consisted of 20 patients, and these were compared to a wait-list group of 20 patients. All three treatments were equally successful in reducing depression with 80 percent of the behavioral treatment group exhibiting a positive response rate.

Teri and Uomoto (1991) presented case studies, using an A-B-A design, that supported the use of a behavioral approach in the treatment of depression with demented elderly. Daily mood ratings of the demented patient by the caregiver were significantly related to the number of pleasant activities in which the demented patient engaged. Depression was substantially reduced in the demented patients by the final week of treatment.

Lewinsohn and Talkington (1979) demonstrated a direct relationship between negative mood and daily aversive events. Daily mood was associated with aversive events over a 30-day period for 146 subjects (r = .29; p<.05). This research led directly to Kanner et al.'s (1981) creation of the Daily Hassles Scale. Hassles were defined as those minor irritations that subjects perceived as troubling. Hassles frequency was highly related to depression in their study of 100 subjects (r = .60; p<.05). Lichtenberg, Swensen, and Skehan (1986) reported a significant relationship between daily hassles and depression in a sample of 70 medically ill elderly (r = .35). Similarly, Lichtenberg and Barth (1990) reported a significant relationship between depression and daily hassles in a sample of 70 caregivers for demented elderly persons (r = .63; p<.05).

Behavioral treatment of depression has a long history of success with older adults, as documented above, and lends itself nicely to adaption to a medical rehabilitation setting. Being hospitalized creates many special circumstances for older adults. There is often a powerful sense of loss and fear over one's future functional status. Hospitals are often impersonal and threatening. Treatments are often aversive, and the pleasant events patients normally engage in are not typically available. The behavioral approach adapted here offers an opportunity to minimize the effects of depression by combating some of the negative consequences that hospitals can produce. It thus offers both theoretical rationale and a practical approach to treatment in a medical setting.

THE DEPRESSION IN OLDER URBAN REHABILITATION PATIENTS TREATMENT PROGRAM: THE DOUR PROJECT

The DOUR project was run coincident with the NSRP studies. Some of the data were shared between the two initiatives, and some samples were unique to one or the other initiatives. Given the shortage of mental health personnel in many medical inpatient settings, the development of treatment protocols involving non-mental health personnel is extremely important. With health care changes increasing the mix of nonprofessional to professional staff, there is a need to expand these types of interventions. Because of the strong evidence that depression affects health outcomes (e.g., functional abilities, mortality), affective disturbance in older patients cannot simply be ignored.

Lichtenberg (1994) reviewed the literature on the use of non-mental health professionals as psychological treatment providers in general, and specifically with regard to older adults. Despite methodological weaknesses in many investigations, such as lack of control groups or objective criteria to measure improvement (see Brown, 1974; Durlak, 1979), the use of non-mental health professionals was supported by dozens of studies. Treatment effectiveness was enhanced when the following criteria were met: (1) there is involvement in a structured behavioral treatment; (2) empathy and warmth are valued characteristics; and (3) there is consistent supervision.

In our treatment study we have emphasized these aspects so as to enhance the likely success of non-mental health professionals in delivering depression treatment. Our protocol is a structured one, based on behavioral theory and methods. Our occupational therapists exhibited interpersonal warmth and empathy, and supervision by the psychologist of treatment was daily.

Hospitalized, medically ill elderly may be especially vulnerable to the lack of pleasurable experiences. Thus, the major tasks of the DOUR project treatment study were to (1) develop a treatment protocol that could be delivered in a medical rehabilitation hospital, (2) specify the treatment in such detail that it could be replicated, and (3) evaluate the effectiveness of the treatment. Because many hospital or rehabilitation settings do not have the requisite number of psychologists to deliver depression treatment, two behavioral treatment protocols were created: (1) treatment delivered by the psychologist and (2) treatment delivered by trained occupational therapists. Participants in these groups were then compared with a no-treatment control group.

Each depression treatment session consisted of (1) relaxation and imagery to reduce anxiety, (2) mood ratings, (3) engaging in a pleasurable event, and (4) positive social praise. A two-step training process was used with the occupational therapists to ensure that treatment procedures were carried out accurately and reliably. First a manual was developed and didactic training was provided based on the manual. Then, after self-study, the therapists practiced the techniques with the PI acting as the depressed patient. The practices were videotaped, and therapists received written and verbal feedback about their performance. A second videotaped practice was undertaken one week later with a nondepressed older adult volunteer acting as the patient. These videotapes were then viewed independently by two expert judges who rated the therapists as to whether they accurately delivered seven observable aspects of treatment. There was 95 percent agreement between the judges, and 95 percent correct delivery of treatment aspects by therapists. At this point, therapists were allowed to engage in the depression treatment.

Procedure

Inclusion criteria: All newly admitted patients were screened within four hours of admission for depression using the Geriatric Depression Scale and Research Diagnostic Criteria for major or minor depression. Depressed subjects (GDS>10), aged 60 or greater, were invited to participate in this study, and their informed consent was obtained. Reevaluation of depression was completed within 24 hours prior to discharge and was always conducted by an interviewer not delivering the treatment. Patients were entered into groups by cohorts. Since most patients interact with one another frequently in a rehabilitation setting, this was done in order that patients in one treatment group would not be exposed to another form of treatment and possibly contaminate the results. The psychology treatment group was entered first, the occupational therapy (interdisciplinary) treatment group was entered next, and the no-treatment group was entered last. All participants signed informed consent documents, and no treatment participants were offered depression treatment as outpatients.

Exclusion criteria: Subjects were adults aged 60 years or older, and were patients admitted to the Rehabilitation Institute of Michigan (RIM) for physical rehabilitation. Patients are most commonly admitted for stroke, orthopedic and other lower extremity disorders, and amputation of the leg. Subjects were excluded from the study if their Mattis Dementia Rating Scale was less than 103 (Mattis, 1988). This score represents the cutoff between mild and moderate dementia (Shay et al., 1991). As described more fully in chapter one, there is a significant relationship between depression and cognition. It was our intent to perform this study on patients with no or mild cognitive problems; nevertheless, the strong relationship between dementia and depression is recognized (see Lichtenberg, 1994). Subjects were excluded from the study if they were on therapeutic doses of antidepressant medication prior to entering the Rehabilitation Institute. The Geriatric Depression Scale scores, and the ADL scores from the Functional Independence Measure were used as criterion measures.

Overview of study: Three groups were included:

- Psychology—received all usual physical and occupational therapies for rehabilitation and depression treatment from a psychologist.
- An occupational therapy group (Interdisciplinary)—received behavioral treatment for depression as part of their occupational therapy sessions and received all usual treatments for physical therapy. They did not receive psychology treatment as part of their rehabilitation.
- No-treatment group—received no depression treatment, but received all usual physical and occupational therapy treatments. Psychology treatment consisted of 30-minute sessions, twice per week.

Occupational therapy treatment sessions were conducted daily, coincident with the functionally based occupational therapy session. Occupational therapists consulted daily with the psychologist in terms of selecting pleasant events, planning positive reinforcement strategies, and receiving support and encouragement. In all, 41 participants were entered into the study, and 37 participants completed the study (13 in psychology treatment, 13 in occupational therapy treatment, and 11 no-treatment controls). The only reasons for participant dropout were acute illness necessitating a readmission to an acute care hospital. The psychology treatment group averaged 4.3 sessions, and the occupational therapy group averaged 7.15 sessions per participant. Of significant note was that most of the depressed patients met the criteria for minor depression only (akin to Blazer's dysphoria group in the 1987 community study). Thus, this population is clearly distinctive from psychogeriatric inpatients.

Results: There was no difference between the groups in terms of age, years of education, cognitive status, severity of comorbid medical diseases, and initial Geriatric Depression Scale score (see Table 3.1). These findings indicate that the three groups were homogeneous and were equivalent on key variables that otherwise might act as moderator variables.

Two 2×3 repeated measures analysis of variances were conducted. Variables evaluated included time (two levels: admit and discharge) and treatment group (three levels: psychology, occupational therapy, no treatment). Post-hoc tests were conducted when the omnibus test result was significant or a trend was found. Table 3.2 is a summary of the results showing that the treatment group depression score improved significantly compared to the no-treatment control group. As can be seen in the table, the time by treatment group interaction was significant ($F = 6.97$; $p<.01$). This means that the rate of change in depression between time 1 and time 2 was dependent upon whether a patient received treatment or did not receive treatment. To illustrate this finding, inspect the mean scores from Table 3.1, which indicated that whereas the treatment groups' depression scores improved, the depression score did not improve in the no-treatment group. Post-hoc analyses indicated that the treatment groups did not differ in reducing depressive symptomatology. Qualitatively, whereas 69 percent of subjects in the two treatment groups showed vast improvements in depression scores, only 25 percent of the no-treatment group improved significantly.

Table 3.3 is a summary of the relationship between ADL skills and depression. In the analysis of variance, there was a trend for the interaction term time by treatment group ($F = 3.09$, $p<.08$). Post-hoc analyses were pursued, and a summary of the one significant result is presented in Table 3.4. As can be seen in Table 3.4, the group that received depression treatment from their occupational therapists improved significantly more with their ADLs than the group that did not receive depression treatment. Qualitatively, whereas over two-thirds of subjects in both treatment groups reached the independent level of functioning for all ADLs, only one-third of the no-treatment group reached independence in all ADLs. Thus, there was partial

TABLE 3.1. Demographic, Medical, ADL, and Depressive Characteristics for Depression Study Subjects

	Psychology Tx	Occupational Therapy Tx	No Tx
Age	78.54 (5.8)	78.69 (6.3)	77.82 (8.2)
Educ.	10.46 (2.3)	10.15 (3.6)	10.36 (3.4)
Sex	10 women, 3 men	13 women	8 women, 3 men
Race	11 A.A., 2 white	12 A.A., 1 white	9 A.A., 2 white
LOS	17.9 (7.7)	12.9 (5.3)	17.4 (5.6)
DRS	123.45 (7.8)	117.83 (14.7)	116.45 (17.2)
GDS1	15.46 (3.3)	16.23 (4.2)	15.55 (4.6)
GDS2	8.92 (4.1)*	10.23 (5.2)*	15.55 (5.4)
CMI	0.92 (1.1)	1.69 (1.1)	1.73 (1.3)
ADL1	29.85 (5.9)	33.00 (4.7)	27.64 (6.7)
ADL2	37.31 (7.3)	42.39 (2.8)*	33.55 (8.5)

Note: *Denotes significantly higher score vs. no-treatment group (p<.01) on one way ANOVAs
Educ.: Years of education
Race: A.A. = African American
LOS: Length of Stay in days
DRS: Mattis Dementia Rating Scale
GDS: Geriatric Depression Scale

TABLE 3.2. 2×3 Repeated Measures Analysis of Variance: Geriatric Depression Scale Scores at Admission and Discharge by Treatment Condition

Source of Variation	SS	DF	MS	F	Sig. F
Within Cells	372.6	34	10.67		
Time	321.2	1	321.2	29.31	.000
Treatment Group by Time	152.8	2	76.42	6.97	.003

TABLE 3.3. 2×3 Repeated Measures Analysis of Variance: Activities of Daily Living Scores at Admission and Discharge by Treatment Condition

Source of Variation	SS	DF	MS	F	Sig. F
Within Cells	276.6	35	7.9		
Time	793.89	1	793.9	100.4	.000
Treatment Group by Time	24.43	1	24.43	3.09	.08

TABLE 3.4. 2×2 Repeated Measures Analysis of Variance Testing: Activities of Daily Living Scores at Admission and Discharge for OT Treatment vs. No-Treatment Conditions

Source of Variation	SS	DF	MS	F	Sig. F
Within Cells	159.0	22	7.23		
Time	696.8	1	696.8	96.42	.000
Treatment Group by Time	35.99	1	35.99	4.98	.03

support for hypothesis 2. Only the group that received depression treatment from occupational therapists improved their ADLs significantly more than the group receiving no depression treatment.

Post-hoc analyses revealed no differences on depression scores and ADL measures between the subjects who received depression treatment from a psychologist and those subjects who received depression treatment from an occupational therapist. Thus, neither method of treatment was superior to the other when outcome measures from the treatment groups were directly compared.

The results of the present study indicate that depression treatment led to improved mood and reduced symptoms of depression, whereas individuals in the no-treatment group did not display improved mood. Inpatient medical rehabilitation involves an intensive period of physical and occupational therapy along with other therapies including intensive rehabilitation nursing care. The emphasis is upon restoration of function and independence. Thus, during routine rehabilitation, patients receive intense individual attention from the health care team members. The results of this study suggest, however, that routine attention alone is not sufficient to improve mood in depressed patients. Depressed patients improved only when they received structured treatment addressing symptoms of depression. Treatment was equally effective when delivered by a psychologist or occupational therapist. The data from the present study provided some limited support for the notion that depression treatment improves functional recovery. Specifically, only treatment delivered through occupational therapy resulted in significant gains in ADLs (even though the no-treatment group received occupational therapy and demonstrated some improvement). The protocol used in this study incorporated functional improvement into the treatment by reinforcing functional progress through verbal praise and graphing. This concrete emphasis on performance may be a required link between reduced depression and improved function. There are several methodological weaknesses that limit the generalizability of this preliminary study. Numbers of subjects per group were small. Follow-up after discharge was not able to be completed, and, thus, the longer term effects (or lack thereof) for treatment could not be determined. The occupational therapists were not blind to the occupational therapy treatment group, and this may have influenced their functional ratings. The possibility of this is mitigated somewhat, however, since the FIM is a highly reliable, behaviorally anchored tool. Nevertheless, the possibility of rater bias existed. Despite these weaknesses, the results of this study appear promising. Late-life depression continues to emerge as a primary health problem, and protocols and data such as these can help ensure that depression is seriously assessed and treated in primary care settings such as hospitals, nursing homes, and physician offices. The unique treatment delivery used here (i.e., occupational therapists as providers of depression treatment) may be one that can be expanded and effectively utilized in these days of reducing health care costs and provider availability.

CLINICAL IMPLICATIONS

Depression, like cognition in the previous chapter, is significantly related to health outcomes. The early recognition and treatment of depression during a medical visit becomes increasingly important when one considers the long-term consequences of depression: worse recovery and higher mortality. While depression is a syndrome and has many potential causes, behavioral treatment can be effectively delivered in medical settings. It may not only reduce the depression, but may increase patients' functional abilities. In those settings where staffing levels allow mental health practitioners to perform the behavioral treatment themselves, psychosocial depression treatment can be a highly productive and visible role on the interdisciplinary team. In those settings where there are not enough mental health practitioners available to deliver treatment, behavioral treatment can be delivered in a collaborative way, with the mental health practitioner supervising the treatment. A specific description of the behavioral treatment of depression is provided in a later chapter.

Chapter 4

Perspectives on Cognition
in Normal Elderly and in Those
with Alzheimer's Disease

LESSONS FOR THE CLINICIAN
FROM STUDIES ON NORMAL AGING

This chapter will be devoted first to reviewing some critical studies on aging and cognition that shed light on aspects that need to be considered when clinicians create and utilize test batteries with older adults. Research methodology will be explored first, followed by a critique of research findings.

CROSS-SECTIONAL AND LONGITUDINAL RESEARCH
CONSIDERATIONS

Research on the effects of age on cognition is conducted in one of two ways: utilizing cross-sectional data or using longitudinal data. Cross-sectional studies refer to the comparison at one point in time of data with persons with characteristics of interest to the researcher. With regard to studies on cognition and aging, cross sectional studies would compare older adults versus younger adults at one point in time. These groups differ in two major ways. Most obvious are the age differences. Less obvious are what is termed cohort differences. A cohort refers to the period of time that an individual was born. If an older adult sample ranged from 70 to 80 years of age, for example, their cohort would consist of those born from 1916 through 1926, whereas a 40- to 50-year-old cohort would consist of those born from 1946 through 1956. Cohort effects refer to the differences between these two groups based solely upon growing up in different eras.

Two interpretations can be made of any positive age-cognition findings in cross-sectional studies. The results may be due to the effects of age, or the results might be due to the effects of cohort (i.e., differences in generations and not due to age). Schaie's (1994) review of his 40 years of research on cognition and aging will be reviewed below to illustrate how cohort and age influence cross-sectional results on cognition and aging. In Schaie's studies, lasting from 1956 to the present, more than 5,000 research subjects from six cohorts completed cognitive testings every seven years. Thus, the study compares cross-sectional and longitudinal data.

By examining the data cross sectionally, linear age declines in cognition were noted in four of six cognitive factors measured. Were these findings due to age or to cohort, or to some of both? By comparing several cohorts and then using longitudinal data, these questions were addressed. Schaie reported that each cohort demonstrated better scores than the previous cohorts on five of the six factors measured. Thus, there was evidence for cohort effects determining some of the linear declines noted on cross-sectional data. Age effects were determined through the use of the longitudinal data.

In contrast to the cross-sectional data, Schaie's longitudinal data on this normal aging sample suggested that there was a linear decline with age only for perceptual speed, and that all cognitive abilities did not reliably decline until after age 67, and then only modest declines were noted. It was only after age 80 that significant declines were noted. The conclusion reached by Schaie was that cross-sectional studies overestimated age-related declines. One final caveat remains, however, and that is the methodological limitations of longitudinal research. Siegler and Botwinick (1979) illustrated the major methodological weakness of longitudinal designs: Subject dropout is not random. Siegler and Botwinick examined 246 subjects aged 60 to 94 years who were participants in a 20-year longitudinal study. Subject attrition from the first to the last testing was progressive and selective. Thus, the sample size declined from 246 at time 1 to 68 at time 5, to 25 by time 10. The mean Full Wechsler Adult Intelligence Scale (WAIS) score from the first testing changed from 85 at the first testing to 115 at the last testing. Clearly, subjects who were performing at a higher level tended to remain in the longitudinal study. Longitudinal studies may thus tend to underestimate age-related changes in cognition.

STUDIES ON MEMORY AND AGING

The relationship between memory functioning and aging has been extensively studied, and has important implications for clinical care. Taylor, Miller, and Tinkenberg (1992) examined the results of 30 subjects ages 60 to 85 who participated in three cognitive testings over a four-year period. The sample consisted of very healthy, very cognitively skilled white subjects (Mean Verbal IQ = 129). The results indicated a 10 percent loss of word recall per year, and a 5 percent loss of perceptual motor speed per year. There was no relationship, however, between word recall and perceptual motor speed, indicating that memory decrements with age may not be a function of decreased speed of perceptual processing.

The stability of decline with increasing age in some aspects of memory functioning and a lack of decline on other aspects of memory functioning has been noted (Verhaegen, Marcoen, and Goosens, 1993; Youngjohn and Crook, 1993). Verhaegen and colleagues performed a meta-analytic study of 40 studies utilizing a number of ways to assess memory (e.g., list recall, paired-associate learning, prose recall). Youngjohn and Crook used everyday memory tests (face-name learning, grocery store list learning) to examine age differences across five age groups. Both studies reported that older adults demonstrated modest effect sizes for decreased acquisition and new learning across all types of memory tasks as compared to middle-aged and young adults. Of more interest, however, is that both studies reported a lack of forgetting, as measured by delayed recall trials. Thus, rate of forgetting may not be related to normal aging, and may be of significance in clinical evaluations. As will be seen later, testing in the memory domain of cognition is the single best discriminator between normal and early dementia subjects. Limitations of these studies, however, also need to be examined. Sampling of less educated and minority populations was limited in these investigations. Thus, it is not known whether these results would be generalizable to older adults in urban settings.

Other Demographic Factors Influencing Cognitive Test Scores

The importance of considering education and other demographic factors was highlighted by recent research (Inouye et al., 1993) in which researchers selected the highest third in terms of physical health and cognitive function and selected them across three cohorts: New Haven, East Boston, and Durham. Even in this highly selected sample, demographic factors predicted large amounts of cognition variance. Whereas education explained 30 percent of cognition score variance, race (African American vs. white) predicted an additional 6 percent of cognition variance above and beyond that accounted for by education. This highlights the importance of norming tests on appropriate samples before applying scores to specific patients. As will be seen, there exist no cognitive test batteries that have utilized a significant number of urban African-American older adults.

CLINICAL IMPLICATIONS FROM NORMAL AGING STUDIES

Clinicians can extract a number of important points from the studies reviewed above. The assessment of cognitive dysfunction is based upon the deficit model. In that model, the patient's scores are compared against performance from a cognitively unimpaired sample who took the same tests. Thus, the accuracy of the clinician's interpretation is to a large extent based upon the quality of their normative data. Interpreting the research on normal aging leads to the following conclusions: Normative data must be roughly equivalent to the patient in age, be from the same cohort, be equivalent in education, and share the same ethnicity. Deviation from these four characteristics may lead to gross errors.

Rate of forgetting is not influenced by age. This is a consistent and pivotal finding for clinicians. Although older adults tend to learn less well than younger adults, once the information is learned they retain the information at the same rate as younger adults. Clinicians who perform memory testing thus should utilize tests of both immediate and delayed recall; to test both learning and rate of forgetting.

DIFFERENTIATING NORMAL AGING FROM DEMENTIA

Dementia is a syndrome, a constellation of symptoms, that has many etiologies. Dementia refers to a decline in cognitive functioning that impedes the affected person's functioning. The most common cause of dementia is Alzheimer's disease. Estimated to affect nearly four million United States citizens, Alzheimer's disease accounts for two-thirds of all dementing illnesses. The certainty of the diagnosis of Alzheimer's disease can only be assured through examination of brain tissue on autopsy. Over the last 15 years, great strides have been made in acquiring brains in which the clinical symptoms of the disease could be compared to the anatomical certainties. Thus, research on Alzheimer's disease is the largest and most advanced research on any of the dementing syndromes and their relationship to cognition. In the material reviewed below, most studies will refer specifically to Alzheimer's disease.

Albert (1981) wrote a seminal paper that continues to serve as a guide for the field of geriatric neuropsychology and the evaluation of cognition through psychometric testing. Albert asserted that the differentiation of cognitive changes associated with normal aging from those changes associated with the beginnings of a pathological process was of chief concern for the field. She cautioned, however, that a range of scores from cognitively unimpaired older adults (i.e., normative data) was severely lacking. She also cautioned that norms based on cross-sectional data would be cohort specific and would need updating with successive cohorts. In the 1990s, normative data on older adults has expanded (Heaton, Grant, and Matthews, 1991; Ivnik et al., 1991; Spreen and Strauss, 1991); however, there are a lack of norms for older adults from urban settings.

Recent evidence has supported the use of psychometric testing in the early identification of pathological cognitive changes in older adults. In a meta-analytic study of 77 reports between 1980 and

1988, memory tests were identified as the best neuropsychological discriminators between demented and nondemented samples (Christensen, Hadzi-Pavlovic, and Jacomb, 1991). Confrontational naming and verbal fluency tasks were also successful discriminators, whereas reading tests were the poorest discriminators. The effect sizes reported by these authors were unrelated to age or to education, but there was no calculation of the impact of culture or race.

Three studies recently investigated the usefulness of psychometric tests of cognition in separating out early dementia from normal functioning. Petersen and colleagues (1994) compared 106 Alzheimer's disease patients with 106 normal patients. The pairs were matched on demographic variables, including age (all subjects were white), and several components of memory were assessed (e.g., free and cued recall, list learning, prose recall, paired associate learning, delayed recall). Other measures included intelligence, attention, and language. Using a logistic regression analysis, memory functioning, specifically acquisition, and number of words recalled over several trials of list learning were the most sensitive in discriminating the two groups, with a 93 percent rate of correct classification. A small subset of 61 subjects, 32 with early Alzheimer's disease, was compared to 29 normal elderly. Once again acquisition was a reliable and significant discriminator between groups.

Becker et al. (1994) conducted a five-year longitudinal study of 204 patients enrolled in an Alzheimer's program. Neuropathologic post mortem examination was conducted with 50 brains, providing definitive diagnoses were able to be definitive for this group of patients. Of the 50 post mortem studies, 43 patients were diagnosed with Alzheimer's disease. Interestingly, accuracy of clinical diagnoses relative to histological inspection was a commendable 86 percent, detailed neuropsychological testing yielded predictive accuracy of 98 percent. Of note, the Mini Mental Status Exam by itself was a poor predictor of diagnoses, accurately identifying only 67 percent of demented individuals. This study provided strong support for somewhat detailed psychometric testing when attempting to identify early dementia in older adults.

In a 13-year prospective study of a community-living, population-based cohort, the development of dementia was tracked and the prediction of dementia onset was studied (Linn et al., 1995). The sample originally consisted of 1,045 subjects aged 65 years or older who were free from dementia at the first cognitive evaluation. During the follow-up period, 55 subjects met the criteria for probable Alzheimer's disease. Cognitive testing consisted of memory, digit span (combined raw score of backward and forward), and verbal fluency tasks (seven tests in all). The average interval between cognitive screening and clinical diagnosis was approximately six years. Although in univariate analyses all neuropsychological measures were associated with the diagnosis of Alzheimer's disease, this was not the case once they controlled for age and education. In the regression equation with age and education controlled, only verbal learning and memory tasks (logical memory immediate and percent retained, paired associate learning) improved the prediction (accounted for additional variance). The authors concluded that indeed a preclinical phase of cognitive deficits is present in Alzheimer's disease for many years before actual diagnosis. Once again, psychometric tests of memory functioning were the best in predicting dementia onset.

A four-year follow-up of the Bronx Aging Study was of particular interest since adults ages 75 to 85, the older old, were targeted (Masur et al., 1994). Initially, 488 nondemented community elders were studied, and 317 completed a yearly evaluation. A two-and-a-half-hour test battery was used, which covered intelligence, learning and memory, verbal fluency, and visuospatial and perceptual motor tasks. Because of the limited age range and the homogeneity of the sample, no demographic predictors of dementia onset were noted. Four tests were able to predict dementia at three times the community-base rate: two aspects of memory, one verbal fluency, and a task of perceptual motor speed.

Clinical Implications

The studies reviewed here, one meta-analytic investigation and four longitudinal studies, present some important converging findings. Despite differences in subject selection (e.g., nondemented community elderly versus elderly seen at an Alzheimer's research program), psychometric test results were among the best markers of early dementia. More specifically, aspects of learning and memory were the most consistent in differentiating between early dementia and normal aging. Clearly, memory testing needs to be a strong component of any dementia test battery.

Methodological Weaknesses of the Studies

There are a number of methodological issues that limit the generalizability of the above findings. The community studies included only very healthy elderly; thus, if they were to become demented, it would likely be due to Alzheimer's disease. Once subjects are excluded because of the presence of hypertension, heart disease, diabetes, or other systemic illnesses, the generalizability to older adults in health care settings is limited. This is particularly true for minority groups such as African-American older adults, who have higher rates of hypertension and diabetes than do white older adults (Pincus and Callahan, 1995). Another limitation of many of the studies is that the subjects were predominantly made up of the young-old. As Schaie's (1994) work points out, there is a significant cognitive decline in normal elderly after age 80. This adds complexity to the clinician's ability to differentiate normal aging from dementia in the oldest-old. Finally, these studies included subjects whose educational level was considerably higher than is found in most urban medical patient groups. As Inouye et al. (1993) reported, education has a large impact on cognitive test scores, even among physically healthy older adults. Nevertheless, the optimistic conclusion of the above studies is that with relatively brief test batteries patients can be well served.

BRIEF COGNITIVE ASSESSMENT BATTERIES

There is a growing awareness of the need for brief psychometric cognitive evaluations, especially in health care settings. First there are cost and reimbursement issues. Many managed care plans limit the length of time they will reimburse for cognitive testing. Second, limited time is also a factor since there is competition for time to perform evaluations, particularly as one competes for time with other interdisciplinary team members (e.g., speech, occupational therapists, physical therapists). Third, there is the issue of fatigue and rapport. Older adults in health care settings fatigue easily, and rapport can be affected dramatically by lengthy (four to eight hours) testing. Finally, there is now empirical support for the use of brief test batteries. The rest of this chapter will be devoted to describing three established brief batteries, and the chapter to follow will introduce the Normative Studies Research Project (NSRP) battery, a brief test battery established on and for use with urban medical patients. Readers will note that two of the three batteries were utilized only with Alzheimer's patients. Research on brief batteries in dementia has focused predominantly on Alzheimer's patients. The three batteries reviewed here are ones that receive the most acclaim.

Washington University Battery

One of the first brief test batteries constructed to document the cognitive effects of dementia was part of a longitudinal study of Alzheimer's disease (Storandt, Botwinick, and Danziger, 1986). The authors utilized portions of the Wechsler Adult Intelligence Scale (WAIS), Wechsler Memory Scale (WMS), the Benton Visual Retention Test, Boston Naming Test, Trailmaking Part A from the Halstead Reitan Battery, Bender Gestalt Test, and Crossing Off Test in their 90- to 120-minute test battery (see Table 4.1 for listing of entire battery). The initial sample included 43 individuals with mild Alzheimer's disease and 43 control subjects enrolled in the Washington University Memory and Aging Project. The subjects were matched on age (mean age was 71 years) and on education (mean education was 12.5 years). Follow-up data, collected over a two-and-a-half-year span, was obtained with 22 of the Alzheimer's subjects and 39 of the control subjects. There were several noteworthy findings from both the cross-sectional and the longitudinal data. First, almost all the tests differentiated the groups initially, including the tests that were hypothesized to be resistant to cerebral deterioration (Information and Comprehension subtests of the WAIS). The Logical Memory subtest of the Wechsler Memory Scale was the most powerful in initially distinguishing between Alzheimer's and control subjects. The only measure that was not useful in dis-

TABLE 4.1. Washington University Battery (1986 to present)

• Wechsler Memory Scale (portions)
• Wechsler Adult Intelligence Scale (portions)
• Benton Visual Retention Test
• Boston Naming Test
• Word Fluency
• Trailmaking Form A
• Bender Gestalt
• Crossing Off Test

tinguishing the groups initially was the Digit Span forward subtest of the WAIS. Examination of the longitudinal data from this study indicated that overall, the Alzheimer's subjects deteriorated over the two-and-a-half-year follow-up period while there was no change in the normal controls.

An outgrowth of this cognitive research was a study to determine whether there is a differential rate of forgetting in Alzheimer's disease subjects versus normal control subjects. Robinson-Whelen and Storandt (1992) compared forgetting rates on the logical memory subtests of the Wechsler Memory Scale, utilizing a 30-minute delay. Sixty-four control subjects were compared to 51 subjects with mild Alzheimer's disease. In a hierarchical regression analysis, immediate recall was a significant predictor of delayed recall, whereas classification as normal or demented was not. Nevertheless, the Alzheimer's subjects retained only 40 percent of the information originally recalled, and the normal subjects retained 70 percent of the information originally remembered.

Using the Washington University battery memory was found to be the most powerful method of discriminating cognitive functioning between normal and demented elderly (Storandt, Botwinick, and Danziger, 1986; Robinson-Whelen and Storandt, 1992). Tests thought to be resistant to dementia were discovered to actually be affected significantly by the dementing condition. A brief testing battery was sufficient to differentiate normal and demented elderly in lieu of the typical six- to eight-hour full neuropsychological test battery.

The Washington University battery has many limits to its generalizability. As described by Storandt, Botwinick, and Danziger (1986), the original sample was comprised of all white, fairly well-educated subjects. Thus, the abilities of these tests to discriminate normal from demented subjects in less educated minority samples was untested.

The Iowa Battery

A comprehensive neuropsychological assessment of normal and demented 60- to 88-year-old adults conducted in Iowa led to the development of a brief 30- to 45-minute battery capable of identifying demented individuals (Eslinger et al., 1985). The original test battery consisted of eight tests (see Table 4.2): four memory tests, one auditory attention task, one verbal fluency task, and two visuospatial tasks. The sample consisted of 53 normal control subjects and 53 dementia subjects matched for age, education, and sex. The means and standard deviations for all tests were significantly higher in the normal subjects than they were in the demented subjects. Certain tests, however, were far better in detecting dementia than were other tests. For example, whereas orientation alone detected dementia in 57 percent of the demented subjects, facial recognition only detected 32 percent.

Stepwise linear discriminant function analyses were used to determine the most effective and parsimonious groups of tests that would detect dementia. Three tests—the Temporal Orientation Test, the Controlled Oral Word Association test, and the Benton Visual

TABLE 4.2. Iowa Battery

- Digit Span
- Logical Memory
- Associate Learning
- Visual Retention
- Word Fluency
- Facial Recognition
- Judgment of Line Orientation

Retention test—were able to accurately classify 85 percent of cases. The authors then cross validated their findings in a new sample of 53 normal and 53 demented individuals. Correct classification, overall, in this sample was 89 percent, providing strong support for the original findings. Limitations of the Iowa battery include its sampling procedures. As with the Washington University battery, there was no mention of minority subjects in the sample.

The CERAD Battery

In 1989, the 16 National Institutes of Health–designated Alzheimer's centers worked together to produce the Consortium to Establish a Registry for Alzheimer's Disease (CERAD) Neuropsychological battery (Morris et al., 1989). The aim of the project was to produce a brief 30- to 40-minute test battery that would characterize the primary manifestations of Alzheimer's disease. Tests were thus chosen to represent aspects of memory, language, and praxis. Tests included a verbal fluency test (animal naming), 15-item Boston Naming test, the full Mini Mental State Exam, a word list memory task that they created, four line drawings, and a word list recognition task that they created (see Table 4.3). Morris and colleagues' 1989 paper described the results from 350 subjects with Alzheimer's disease, and 275 control subjects. Test-retest reliability correlations over a one-month period ranged from .52 to .78. The tests readily distinguished normal controls from Alzheimer's patients. The authors interpreted these data as providing solid support for the CERAD battery. Methodological weaknesses included having a younger and more highly educated control group than patient group, and inclusion of few minority subjects.

TABLE 4.3. CERAD Battery

• Verbal Fluency (Animal category)
• 15-item Boston Name Test
• MMSE
• Word List Memory
• Four Line Drawings
• Word List Recognition

Subjects matched for sex, age, and education were utilized in the next investigation of the utility of the CERAD battery (Welsh et al., 1991). One hundred ninety-six subjects were placed into one of four groups: a control group, a mildly demented group, a moderately demented group, and a severely demented group. The average age of the subjects was 71 years, and the average education was 14 years. Stepwise linear discriminant function analysis was utilized to determine how accurately the CERAD battery classified subjects. Ninety-six percent of both the normal controls and the moderately and severely demented group were classified accurately, and 86 percent of the mild group was accurately classified. The best predictor was the delayed recall score from the word list. The percent retained dropped from 85.6 percent in the normal controls, to 35.8 percent in the mildly impaired group, to 16 percent in the moderate and severely impaired group. The worst predictors were the number of intrusion errors on the word list recall and recognition tasks, and the recognition memory score. The authors concluded that the CERAD battery may be useful in aiding in the early detection of dementia. Limitations of this study were similar to those found in the other studies mentioned previously. This sample utilized a relatively well-educated white sample and had a relatively young sample (mean was 71 years, standard deviation 5 years).

A normative study of the CERAD conducted by Welsh and her colleagues (1994) utilized 413 white subjects who were recruited from 23 sites across the United States. Subjects were divided into those who completed at least a high school education and those who completed less than a high school education. Few subjects in this lower education group did not have at least some high school experience. In the more highly educated group, there were age effects found for performance on memory tests, whereas no age effects were found for the less educated group. Of special note was that the savings score (i.e., the number of words remembered during the delayed recall trial expressed as a percentage of what was originally remembered on the last trial of the immediate recall of the word list) on the delayed word list recall task was unaffected by age. Savings score represents the amount of material retained between original learning and a delayed recall task. It is important to remember that studies of normal aging demonstrated that there was equal retention of learned information between older and younger adults (i.e., savings score). This is important, the authors concluded, because savings scores are often among the best indicators of early dementia.

The CERAD battery research presents many impressive findings, particularly a high degree of accuracy in classification while utilizing a brief set of test procedures. A number of methodological limitations limit the generalizability and clinical utility of these findings, however. The only demented group of study was Alzheimer patients who attend a designated Alzheimer's center. Thus, the usefulness of this test battery in a general geriatric neuropsychology practice such as a healthcare setting is unknown. Would this battery be sensitive to decline due to vascular dementia or to dementia due to alcohol abuse or due to other etiologies? The current lack of application of the CERAD battery to this group severely limits its uses currently.

Unverzagt et al. (1996) published the first normative data on African Americans who reside in an urban area. Their findings illustrate the importance of understanding the limits of generalizability of normative data sets. Eighty-three subjects, completing a mean of nine years of education, demonstrated reduced scores on the CERAD Boston Naming and memory tests as compared to previous normative samples made up of more highly educated, white older adults. Factor analysis of the Unverzagt sample yielded a two-factor solution: a memory factor and a general intellectual functioning factor. The clinical utility of the CERAD in an urban population of older adults remains unknown, however, since no patient data was gathered.

Although there are other brief test batteries used to assess dementia, none have been utilized in widespread fashion. A listing of some of the other brief batteries not reviewed here, nevertheless, are noted in Table 4.4. These batteries have not received the widespread interest or in-depth study as have the three batteries reviewed earlier.

Clinical Implications

The studies summarized above provide clear guidance as to the clinical utility of brief cognitive test batteries in working with older adults. Data on differentiating demented from nondemented elderly

TABLE 4.4. Listing of Other Brief Batteries

- Alzheimer's Disease Assessment Scale
- Cognitive Battery for Dementia
- Telephone Interview for Cognitive Status
- Test for Severe Impairment
- Neuropsychological Screening Battery

point to the importance of emphasizing memory assessment in the cognitive evaluation. Indeed, memory functioning was a key test in each of the brief batteries reviewed. Tasks of attention, language, visuospatial functioning, and executive functioning, as well as general tests of cognitive functioning, were all clinically useful in the identification of demented individuals. Reading tests, in contrast, provide useful information because they are relatively poor at discriminating between demented and nondemented individuals. Reading tests can be used as crude estimates of an individual's premorbid level of intellectual functioning. The data on brief batteries provides support for the notion that cognitive assessment of older adults can be completed in a timely, cost-effective fashion without sacrificing diagnostic accuracy.

A test battery must be established to help guide the assessment of cognition in older medical patients. Limitations of the research reviewed in this chapter were the sole focus on Alzheimer's patients and the limited information available on urban, medically ill individuals. In the next chapter, a test battery will be described that was created for the assessment of cognition in medically ill urban elderly. Consistent with the research presented in this chapter, the battery will be brief (one to two hours), and will utilize tests that tap into a variety of cognitive domains known to be sensitive to dementia. In addition to normative data, clinical utility data will also be presented.

Defining a normative group among medical patients is a complex issue. Diseases such as uncontrolled diabetes, hypertension, and pulmonary disease are known to have effects on cognition (Tarter, Van Thiel, and Edwards, 1988). Thus, stringent inclusion criteria were utilized in each data set for the NSRP. First, patients were required to demonstrate unimpaired performance on a performance-based measure of general cognitive functioning as defined by scoring in the independent range on the FIM cognition items, and scoring within one standard deviation of the mean using published norms on the Dementia Rating Scale (except when the DRS was being studied, then Logical Memory I was used). Second, patients were independent in all of their activities of daily living. These included grooming, bathing, feeding, toileting, transferring, eating, and dressing. Finally, patients had no neurologic diagnoses as assessed by their attending physicians.

Chapter 5

The Normative Studies Research Project Test Battery

NSRP GOALS

The Normative Studies Research Project (NSRP) was designed to develop normative data and to examine the clinical utility of particular neuropsychological tests. The unique aspects of this work were the samples that were utilized. As described earlier in this book, an older urban medical population was used. Compared to most normative samples, then, the NSRP research projects included more individuals with less than a high school education, and more minority subjects. The NSRP began by first investigating individual tests. The NSRP test battery was only developed later, after several years of utilizing a variety of different measures. In this chapter, the research on the individual tests studied will be highlighted and then followed by a review of the complete NSRP test battery, as well as research related with the test battery.

Research has investigated six tests in depth. These will be reviewed here, with an emphasis on describing the relationship of test scores to demographic factors, and the provision of normative data for the urban medical population that we worked with. In Table 5.1 are listed descriptions of the NSRP study samples. Because the NSRP test battery was only developed in full after several years of practice, some samples are much larger than others. As can be seen in the table, for example, the full NSRP test battery study included 237 patients, whereas the Logical Memory subtests study utilized 343 patients.

TABLE 5.1. Sample Characteristics of NSRP Normative Studies

Study	Size	Description
Nabors, Vangel, Lichtenberg, and Walsh (in press)	N = 117	Consecutively tested older patients who received Hooper Visual Organization Test.
Lichtenberg, Ross, Youngblade, and Vangel (n.d.)	N = 237	Consecutively tested older patients who received all core NSRP tests.
Lichtenberg, Ross, and Christensen (1994)	N = 57	Consecutively tested older patients who received Boston Naming Test.
Ross, Lichtenberg, and Christensen (1995) Kimbarow, Vangel, and Lichtenberg (1996)	N = 274	Consecutively tested older patients (includes the 57 from earlier study) who received Boston Naming Test.
Lichtenberg, Millis, and Nanna (1994)	N = 61	Consecutively tested older patients who received Visual Form Discrimination Test.
Nabors, Vangel, and Lichtenberg (1996)	N = 184	Consecutively tested older patients (includes the 61 from the earlier study) who received the Visual Form Discrimination Test.

GENERAL COGNITION: MATTIS DEMENTIA RATING SCALE

The Dementia Rating Scale (Mattis, 1988) was initially constructed to assess the general cognitive abilities of demented patients. A broad range of functions including attention, language, memory, reasoning, and construction tasks were included in the scale. In a study of 30 demented patients, Coblentz and colleagues (1973) provided good evidence for test-retest reliability (r = .97) and concurrent validity between the Dementia Rating Scale and the WAIS IQ score (r = .75). An estimate of split-half reliability was found to be in the adequate range as well (r = .90) by Gardner et al. (1981). Vitaliano and colleagues (1984) found that the Dementia Rating Scale significantly differentiated between normal, mildly demented, and moderately to severely demented patients.

Initial norms for the DRS were provided by Coblentz and colleagues (1973), using a sample of 11 healthy adults of average intelligence, all of whom scored above 140 on the DRS. Montgomery and Costa (1983) derived norms from 85 community dwellers with an age range of 65 to 81. This group had a mean DRS total score (DRS-T) of 137 and a standard deviation of 6.9. A cutoff score was established at 123 (-2 SD). Schmidt et al. (1994) derived norms from 1,001 Austrian subjects with an age range of 50 to 80, who were participants in a stroke prevention program. This sample was stratified by age and education, with means ranging from 139 to 143. Normative samples from the United States have been relatively ethnically homogeneous and highly educated, and no study of the relationship of DRS-T and demographic characteristics has been done. Most importantly, no data exist, for any sample, on individuals older than 81 years.

Two studies support the utility of the DRS for discriminating levels of impairment. Vitaliano and colleagues (1984) found significant differences on DRS-T between control subjects and mildly impaired and moderately impaired Alzheimer's patients. Shay and colleagues (1991) found DRS-T to classify 100 percent of moderately impaired Alzheimer's patients as impaired, with 71 percent classified within the moderately impaired group and 29 percent within the mildly impaired group.

Our study had two purposes: first, to examine the relationship of DRS-T to demographic variables, including age; and second, to derive norms and discriminability data for urban medical inpatients, based on preestablished impairment rating groups (Vangel and Lichtenberg, 1995). Subjects included 56 males and 139 females. Sixty-four were Caucasian and 131 were African American. The mean age was 77, with a standard deviation of 7 and a range from 62 to 95. Mean education was 9.8 years, with a standard deviation of 3.7 and a range of 1 to 21 years. Subjects' primary diagnoses included 79 fractures, 60 musculoskeletal disorders, 38 abnormalities of gait, 23 neurological disorder, 11 coma, 2 circulatory disease, and 2 decreased coordination.

Ninety patients met all three criteria for inclusion in the intact group. These included independence with all ADLs, no neurological diagnoses, and scoring within one standard deviation of the mean Logical Memory I score. The group had a mean age of 74 and standard deviation of 5.9. Twenty-four were males and 66 were female. Fifty-three were African American, 36 Caucasian. Mean education was 10.5 years, with a standard deviation of 3.6.

Cognitively intact patients were divided into two subgroups for some analyses: 79 and younger and 80 and above. The groups were split at these age breakings so as to allow direct comparisons with previous norms that only went up to age 79. The 73 patients of the younger group had a mean age of 72.3, with a standard deviation of 4.0, and a mean education of 10.6, with a standard deviation of 3.7. The 17 patients of the older group had a mean age of 83.5, with a standard deviation of 2.9, and a mean education of 10.3, with a standard deviation of 3.1. The impaired group had a lower mean educational level (M = 9.2, SD = 3.8) and a higher mean age (M = 79, SD = 7) than did the cognitively intact group.

Pearson and point biserial correlations of demographic measures and DRS-T for the cognitively intact group are presented in Table 5.2. DRS-T significantly correlated with age (r = -.28, p < .01) and education (r = .24, p < .05), such that older participants scored more poorly on the DRS, and those with more reported years of education had higher DRS scores. DRS-T was not significantly correlated with race or gender. Additionally, both age (t(192.85) = -5.42, p < .001) and education (t(190.83) = 2.57, p < .05) were significantly different across impairment rating groups.

TABLE 5.2. Pearson and Point Biserial Correlations of DRS Score with Demographics for the Cognitively Intact Group (n = 90)

	Age	Race	Gender	Education	DRS
Age	—				
Race	−.03	—			
Gender	.11	−.06	—		
Education	−.13	.10	.09	—	
DRS	−.28**	.15	.14	.24*	—

Note: *p <.05, **p <.01

Gender, race, age, and education were entered as a block in a stepwise multiple regression analysis. The model met assumptions of normality and freedom from collinearity, but slight heteroskedasticity was present. The model accounted for 17 percent of DRS-T variance ($F(85,4) = 3.93, p < .01$). Of the four predictors, only age had significant unique variance in the prediction of DRS-T ($ß = -.27$, $p < .05$). Although both age and education were correlated with DRS-T, the relationship of education to the DRS-T can be accounted for in terms of age.

The cognitively intact group had a mean DRS total score (DRS-T) of 132.8, with a standard deviation of 6.9. As can be seen in Table 5.3, there were differences on the DRS between the younger and older groups. The older group scored lower on the DRS memory subscale, thus producing a lower mean and greater standard deviation on the DRS-T as compared to the younger group. Table 5.4 presents a comparison of the mean scores reported by Mattis (1988) and those found in our study. For the younger group, the means and standard deviations between the Mattis norms and our own were virtually identical. The mean DRS was lower, however, for the older group.

The clinical utility of the DRS was assessed by logistic regression analysis. Eighty-seven percent of cases were correctly classified into intact or impaired groups based on DRS-T. Correct classification rates were 89 percent for the intact group and 86 percent for the impaired group. Z for the probability of membership in the impaired group ($1 / 1 + e^{-Z}$) is equal to the linear combination of logistic regression coefficients $= 20.0158 + .0581(age) - .1961 (DRS-T)$). Age was not a significant predictor of impairment ($R = .07$, Wald $= 3.24, p > .05$). The addition of DRS-T resulted in a significant increase in predictability ($R = -.39$, Wald $= 42.11, p < .0001$. DRS-T was negatively related to assignment in the impaired group.

A DRS-T cutting score of 120, being close to two standard deviations from the mean DRS-T for the intact group, resulted in a correct classification of 84 percent overall, with a sensitivity of 74 percent and a specificity of 93 percent. A second cutting score (DRS-T $= 125$) was selected to maximize overall correct classification at 87 percent, with 85 percent sensitivity and 90 percent specificity. Similar classification rates were found for the younger

TABLE 5.3. Intact Group Means and Standard Deviations of DRS Scores for Two Age Ranges

	Age Ranges	
DRS Scales	**62 - 79** **(n = 73)**	**80 - 95** **(n = 17)**
Total Score	M = 133.8 SD = 6.3	M = 128.2 * SD = 8.2
Attention	M = 35.3 SD = 1.3	M = 35.1 SD = 2.0
Initiation/Preservation	M = 33.9 SD = 3.3	M = 31.7 SD = 4.9
Construction	M = 5.5 SD = 1.3	M = 5.1 SD = 1.8
Conceptualization	M = 35.5 SD = 2.8	M = 34.7 SD = 2.8
Memory	M = 23.4 SD = 1.8	M = 20.7 * SD = 3.5

Note: * significant difference between age groups ($p < .05$)

TABLE 5.4. Normative Observations for Older Adults Using the Mattis Dementia Rating Scale: Effects of Age

Author of Norms	**Mean Age**	**Mean Education**	**DRS Total**
Mattis (1988)	74 (6)*	unknown	137.3 (7)
Vangel and Lichtenberg (1995)	72 (4)	10.6 (3)	133.8 (6)
Vangel and Lichtenberg (1995)	83 (3)	10.6 (3)	128.2 (8)
Sample sizes			
Mattis (n = 82)			
Vangel and Lichtenberg	(young-old n = 73) (old-old n = 17)		

Note: * Standard deviations are listed in parentheses.

and older age groups when using cut-off scores of 125 and 123, respectively. It was concluded that the DRS is a good screening instrument for this population, although extreme care must be utilized when interpreting scores of those over age 80, particularly if they report few years of education.

MEMORY: LOGICAL MEMORY SUBTEST OF THE WECHSLER MEMORY SCALE–REVISED (WMS–R)

The Logical Memory (LM) subtest (I and II) consists of two paragraph-length stories that are read to the patient. Logical Memory I is the patient's immediate recall of the stories. The total bits of information recalled by the patient from story 1 and story 2 are added together to give the Logical Memory I score. Logical Memory II is a delayed recall task. Thirty minutes after Logical Memory I is administered, patients are asked to recall the stories as best they can. Thus, there are three scores derived from this test. An immediate recall score (LMI), a delayed recall score (LMII), and a savings score as represented by the proportion of LMI recalled during LMII. Savings scores were reviewed in the previous chapter and were noted to be unchanged during normal aging, and to being especially sensitive to discriminating between demented and cognitively intact older adults.

While there is a lack of normative data on the Logical Memory subtest in the WMS-R manual (Wechsler, 1987), four recent studies provided such normative data for older adults (Cullum et al., 1990; Ivnik et al., 1992; Lichtenberg and Christensen, 1992). A fifth study expanded on the Lichtenberg and Christensen study and explored the norms and clinical utility of the Logical Memory subtest in an older urban sample of mostly African-American medical patients (Vangel, Lichtenberg, and Ross, in press).

Early studies on the Logical Memory subtests have found good evidence for their clinical utility. Savings scores, for example, were used to differentiate normals from each of three clinical groups: amnestics, Alzheimer's patients, and Huntington's disease patients, and also discriminated the clinical groups from each other (Butters et al., 1988; Troster et al., 1993).

Three hundred forty-three patients, 99 cognitively intact and 245 cognitively impaired, comprised our NSRP sample. The intact group had a mean age of 75 years (SD = 6.7) and a mean educational level of 10.8 (SD = 3.4). Seventy-one percent were female and 60 percent were African American. The impaired group had the same ethnic composition as the intact group but were slightly older (M = 78.2, SD = 7.5) and less educated (M = 9.8, SD = 3.4) than the intact group.

In Table 5.5 are the intercorrelations between demographic variables and the Logical Memory subtest measures. Age had significant correlations with LMI (r = -.17; p<.05) and LMII (r = -.27; p<.05), whereas education had a significant correlation only with LMI (r = .27; p<.05). Thus, older, less educated patients performed more poorly on LMI than did younger, better educated patients. Age alone was related to LMII scores, with older patients scoring lower when compared to younger patients. Age and education were significantly correlated with each other (r = -.21; p<.05), indicating that the oldest patients completed fewer years of education than did the younger patients. Race and gender were unrelated to LMI or LMII scores, and no demographic variable was correlated with savings score.

Hierarchical multiple regression analysis results revealed that demographic factors accounted for only 9 percent of LMI variance and 8 percent of LMII variance. Education was the only unique

TABLE 5.5. Pearson and Point Biserial Correlations of Test Scores and Demographics for the Cognitively Intact Group (n = 99)

	LM I	LM II	Savings	DRS
Age	−.17*	−.27*	−.13	.09
Race	−.04	−.02	−.10	.19*
Gender	.06	−.02	−.10	.23*
Education	.27*	.15	−.07	.22*
LM I	—	.77**	−.27*	.47*
LM II	—	—	.19*	.45**
Savings	—	—	—	−.12

Note: * p < .05
      ** p < .01

predictor of LMI, whereas age was the only unique predictor of LMII. The means and standard deviations reported in Table 5.6 for the cognitively intact are slightly lower than those reported by Ivnik and colleagues (1992), and much lower than those reported by Cullum and his colleagues (1990) (see Table 5.7).

Discriminant Function Analyses (DFA) were carried out to investigate how well the cognitively intact and cognitively impaired groups could be correctly classified based on LM scores. For LMI, a significant discriminant function was found (Wilks = .891, F = 41.8; p<.05), but only 67 percent of cases overall were correctly classified. Specificity was at 65 percent and sensitivity was at 69 percent. The DFA was significant for LMII (Wilks = .852, F = 59.5; p<.05), correctly classifying 73 percent of cases overall. Specificity was a low 31 percent, whereas sensitivity was 90 percent. Using a cutoff score at the .85 specificity level, LMI = 10 was identified (sensitivity was .46 at that cut score). For LMII, a cutoff score at .85 specificity was identified as LMII = 6 (sensitivity was .52 at that cut score). Finally, at the .85 specificity level, 53 percent was identified as a savings cut score (sensitivity was .48 at this score).

Two major conclusions were drawn from these data. The LM normative data provided here may be more applicable to older ethnically diverse urban medical patients than are previous norms. Second, practitioners need be aware of the relatively poor discriminability found with the LM subtests in this sample. It is recommended, therefore, that conservative cutoff scores be used, and that

TABLE 5.6. Means and Standard Deviations of Test Scores for Cognitively Intact and Cognitively Impaired Subjects

	Intact		Impaired	
	Mean	**s.d.**	**Mean**	**s.d.**
LM I	16.6	5.9	11.8	6.3*
LM II	12.9	6.3	7.2	6.3*
Savings	86%	8%	57%	5%*
DRS Total	133.5	4.9	115.4	14.9

Note: *Significant difference between intact and impaired groups (p .05).

TABLE 5.7. Normative Comparisons for Older Adults Using the Logical Memory Subtests of the Wechsler Memory Scale–Revised

Author of Norms	Mean Age	Mean Education	LMI	LMII
Cullum et al. (1990)	79.8 (4)*	14.6 (3)	25.0 (7)	20.9 (8)
Lichtenberg and Christensen (1992)	77.3 (6)	11.3 (3)	17.8 (6)	13.7 (6)
Ivnik et al. (1992)	79	12	19-21	14-15

Sample Sizes

Cullum et al. (n = 32)

Lichtenberg and Christensen (n = 66)

Ivnik et al. (n = 441)

Note: *Standard deviations are listed in parentheses.

LM subtests be used along with other memory measures when assessing cognitive function in urban elderly medical patients.

FULD OBJECT MEMORY EVALUATION

The Fuld Object Memory Evaluation (OME) was developed to evaluate different component abilities of memory functioning (e.g., storage and retrieval) in the elderly. The OME uses a procedure that attempts to limit the effects of hearing and vision impairments upon test performance. It forces the individual being evaluated to cognitively process the information to be remembered by tactually recognizing the object, visually recognizing the object, naming it, and then, if still unable to identify the object, hearing the name of it (Fuld, 1980). After ensuring patients have cognitively processed the stimuli to be remembered, they are asked to recall the objects after a distraction period on each of five trials. After each trial, patients are selectively reminded of items not recalled. The Fuld OME produces scores on four indices: storage, retrieval, repeated retrieval, and ineffective reminders. Two are indices of retrieval skills (i.e., retrieval and repeated retrieval) whereas two are indices of storage (i.e., storage and ineffective reminders).

The original normative data (Fuld, 1980) were provided by a sample of high-achieving, cognitively intact elderly white members of a senior citizen's center. Cognitively intact and impaired subjects were matched on age, country of birth, and occupational achievement. The final sample consisted of 15 70- to 79-year-old intact individuals and 17 80- to 89-year-old intact individuals.

Other studies have found the OME to be useful in differentiating primary degenerative dementia from depression or other organic disorders (LaRue, 1989; LaRue et al., 1986). In those studies, LaRue and her colleagues reported that the OME better discriminated the three groups than did the Benton Visual Retention Test (Used in the Iowa Battery) and a paired associate learning test. Finally, in the Masur et al. (1994) study mentioned earlier, in which dementia onset was measured prospectively, the Fuld OME was one of the best predictors of dementia onset.

One hundred fifty subjects total comprised our NSRP normative data and clinical utility study (Summers, Lichtenberg, and Vangel, 1995). Sixty-three subjects comprised the cognitively intact group, with a mean educational level of 10.5 years (SD = 3.1) and a mean age of 77 years (SD = 5.1). Two-thirds of the group were African Americans and 73 percent of the group were women. Ninety-two participants belonged to the cognitively impaired group. This group had the same ethnic makeup of the intact group, but were significantly older (M = 79 years, SD = 5.0) and less educated (M = 9.1, SD = 3.8) than the intact group.

Intercorrelations between the Fuld OME indices and demographic variables for our intact group can be found in Table 5.8. Age was significantly correlated with each index on the OME, with correlations ranging from −.39 to −.48. No other demographic variable (i.e., education, race, sex), however, was significantly correlated with any Fuld indice. When multiple regression analyses were used, 20 to 26 percent of variance was accounted for by age on each of the Fuld indices.

TABLE 5.8. Intercorrelations of Demographic Variables and OME Indices for the Cognitively Intact Group

	1	2	3	4	5	6	7	8
1. Age	—							
2. Education	.05	—						
3. Gender	−.08	−.07	—					
4. Race	.06	.09	.07	—				
5. Retrieval	−.46**	−.12	.05	−.15	—			
6. Storage	−.39**	−.14	.13	−.14	.80**	—		
7. Repeated Retrieval	−.48**	−.08	−.01	−.15	.96**	.64**	—	
8. Ineffective Reminders	.41**	.13	−.13	.12	−.87**	−.84**	−.74**	—

Note: * $p < .05$
** $p < .01$

In Table 5.9 are the means and standard deviations of scores from our cognitively intact sample and from the original normative sample by Fuld. The scores from our sample were almost identical to those reported by Fuld. Both studies found clear differences between age groups with the older subjects (80 to 89 years) scoring lower than the 70- to 79-year-old group.

The clinical utility of the Fuld OME was examined by use of a Discriminant Function Analysis. Overall classification was 75 percent, with a specificity of 85 percent and a sensitivity of 68.5 percent. Further investigation of sensitivity and specificity of the Fuld OME was obtained by using a cutoff score of one standard deviation below the mean for the cognitively intact group. In the 70- to 79-year-old group, specificity ranged from a high of 91 percent (storage index) to a low of 79 percent (repeated retrieval). Sensitivity ranged from a high of 67 percent (retrieval) to a low of 57 percent (storage). In the 80- to 89-year-old group specificity was 85 percent in three indices and 90 percent for the storage indice. Sensitivity ranged from 72 percent to 63 percent.

TABLE 5.9. Normative Observations on the Fuld Object Memory Evaluation for Older Adults

Author of norms	Storage	Retrieval	RR	IR
Age group 1: 70-79				
Fuld (1977)	45.7 (2)*	38.7 (4)	25.8 (5)	2.1 (2)
Summers, Lichtenberg, and Vangel (1995)	44.5 (3)	37.6 (4)	23.8 (5)	2.8 (3)
Age group 2: 80-89				
Fuld (1977)	40.8 (6)	33.6 (6)	21.0 (5)	6.3 (5)
Summers and Lichtenberg (1994)	42.5 (3)	33.9 (6)	20.0 (6)	5.4 (4)
Sample sizes				

Fuld   (70-79 n = 15)
        (80-89 n = 17)

Summers and Lichtenberg (70-79 n = 43)
                         (80-89 n = 20)

Note: *Standard deviations are listed in parentheses.

The results led to conflicting conclusions. On the one hand, the Fuld OME holds up well, since the scores from our sample were identical to those of the original normative sample, which used more highly educated individuals. On the other hand, the Fuld OME has a relatively low ceiling, and sensitivity is poor since even impaired patients may perform well on the test. Still, if an individual performs poorly on the OME, there is a good chance the person is experiencing significant memory deficits.

LANGUAGE: BOSTON NAMING TEST

Decreased language functioning, particularly naming abilities, are often early symptoms of central nervous system diseases such as cortical dementia and other degenerative disorders (Heilman and Valenstein, 1993). Thus, knowledge of age-related performance on naming tasks for elderly individuals is essential in order to discriminate between normal aging and a dementing process. The Boston Naming Test (BNT) (Kaplan, Goodglass, and Weintraub, 1983) is an established clinical tool for assessing naming deficits associated with a variety of neuropathological conditions. Originally published with 85 items (Kaplan, Goodglass, and Weintraub, 1978), the present 60-item version is a commonly used psychometric test in assessing some aspects of language functioning. Patients are presented with pictures of objects that they are then asked to name. If they cannot name the object, patients are given a clue (e.g., an ocean animal for octopus). If they still cannot name the object, they fail the item.

Studies using the Boston Naming Test to detect the effects of aging on naming abilities have generally found decreases, particularly beyond the eighth decade of life. Three studies reported on the effects of aging on Boston Naming Test scores using the 85-item version of the test, while two utilized the 60-item version. In their sample of 80 optimally healthy older adults, Albert, Heller, and Milberg (1988) reported a significant correlation of $r = -.39$ with age. Nicholas and colleagues (1985) and Labarge, Edwards, and Knesevich (1986) also found modest naming decrements with advancing age. In their samples of highly educated, optimally healthy older adults, Mitrushina and Satz (1989) and VanGorp and colleagues (1986) found modest, significant relationships between age and naming on the 60-item test with correlation coefficients of $r = -.29$ and $r = -.33$, respectively. In these two samples, the mean scores varied by only five points between those aged 57 to 65 and those over age 80, although the variance did increase with age. Thus, the normative data presented and suggested cutoff scores change little with advancing age.

Normative data for the 60-item Boston Naming Test with the elderly is limited in two ways. First, the strongest normative data on the elderly (i.e., VanGorp et al., 1986) used a more highly educated group of older adults than is generally found in most clinical practice. The 24 individuals used in this study were between the ages of 70 and 74 and had a mean education level of 15.25 years and a mean Verbal IQ of 130. In both Mitrushina and Satz (1989) and VanGorp et al.'s (1986) samples, the mean level of education was two years of college. Second, there has been no investigation of the effects of ethnicity on Boston Naming Test scores in the elderly. Are there differences, for example, between scores for cognitively intact older white and African-American patients?

We focused upon three main areas of research in the NSRP investigation of the BNT: (1) Relationship of demographic variables to BNT test scores and the establishment of norms for older, less-educated whites and African Americans in urban settings; (2) A focus on investigating which of the items were most influenced by ethnicity; and (3) An investigation of the clinical utility of the BNT. The main aspects of each of these studies will be reviewed.

Lichtenberg, Ross, and Christensen (1994) investigated the relationship between demographic variables and BNT scores in 57 cognitively intact older adults (29 African American, 28 White; 31 women, 26 men). Overall, the group had a mean educational level of 11.2 years (SD = 3.2 years). Correlational analyses showed that scores on the Boston Naming Test (n = 57) were unrelated to education (r = .08) or gender (r = -.09). Consistent with previous research, a significant but modest negative correlation was found between age and Boston Naming Test score (r = -.42; p<.001). A significant relationship was found between ethnicity and the Boston Naming Test (r = .26; p = .05), indicating that whites performed better than did African Americans. A 2×3 analysis of variance was performed in order to further determine the relationship between Boston Naming Test scores and age and ethnicity. Main effects were found for both age (F = 4.4; p = .017) and ethnicity (F = 4.7; p = .035). Overall, the variables accounted for 21 percent of the variance. No significant interaction effects were found (F = .30; p = .74). Table 5.10 lists the means, standard deviations, and suggested cutoff scores for the Boston Naming Test among three age groupings and calculated for African Americans and whites. Cutoff scores of two standard deviations were chosen.

An inspection of the data revealed two things. First, the greater variance among the African-American subjects make the cutoff scores for this group much lower than for the white subjects. Second, when compared to VanGorp and colleagues' group, the cutoff scores for the entire NSRP sample are considerably lower. For example, the cutoff scores for their 75 to 79 and over-80 group are

TABLE 5.10. Normative Data on the BNT for a Group of Normal Older Adults

		BNT Scores		
Group	n	M	SD	Suggested Cutoff*
1. 70 to 74 Years Old	22	47.32	9.52	
African American	12	46.00	11.55	23
White	10	48.90	6.15	37
2. 75 to 79 Years Old	20	42.95	8.76	
African American	8	38.75	9.21	20
White	12	45.75	7.57	30
3. 80+ Years Old	15	38.80	8.89	
African American	8	36.00	9.44	17
White	7	42.00	7.62	26

Note: *Cutoff scores were computed for two standard deviations below the mean as VanGorp et al. (1986) suggested.

not even one standard deviation below the mean scores for the white subjects in this sample. For African-American subjects, the cutoff scores are even more disparate as compared to previous norms. The mean score for the African-American sample of persons over 80 years old, for example, is lower than the cutoff in VanGorp et al.'s sample.

In our next study, we doubled the sample and investigated the same questions (Ross, Lichtenberg, and Christensen, 1995). One hundred twenty-three subjects, 72 African Americans and 51 whites with a mean age of 75.87 (SD = 7.4 years) years and a mean educational level of 11 years (SD = 3.4 years) were studied. Correlations in this sample revealed that age, education, and race were significantly related to BNT score. Indeed, when entered together in a multiple regression analysis, the three variables accounted for 37 percent of BNT variance. Subsequent regression analyses revealed that each demographic variable predicted unique BNT variance, above and beyond that accounted for the other two variables (Kimbarow, Vangel, and Lichtenberg, 1996).

In Table 5.11 are listed the norms developed on this second, larger study. These norms are broken out only by age, and thus samples of 40 or greater are found for each age group. The norms published by Van Gorp and Mitushina are also found in Table 5.11.

The influences of demographic data were further studied through the process of item analysis (Kimbarow, Vangel, and Lichtenberg, 1996). This study used the exact same sample as the Ross study cited above. Based on the percentage correct in the overall sample, items were grouped into three categories of 20 items each, ranging from relatively high correct percentages (i.e., 95 to 100 percent) to relatively low ones (4 to 40 percent). A total score of correct responses was summed for each group, and African American and white subjects were compared. Scores having modest difficulty were the ones that best separated the groups, with whites identifying more correct responses than did African Americans. This grouping of 20 items included such items to be named as octopus, pretzel, snail, canoe, igloo. In Table 5.12 the items are broken down into the three groups (easiest to hardest). As can be seen in the table, there are some discrepancies between the ease of items and the order in which they are presented. For example, items 13, 19, 46, and 49 were found to be of modest difficulty. Two of these items are in the first third of the test, while the other two are in the last third. At this point, it is difficult to know how to use these data in clinical practice, although they reemphasize the need to be conservative in clinical interpretation.

The differences on the BNT between whites and African Americans are likely a function of cultural differences that may even be unique to this cohort. A majority of our African-American patients were raised in the rural south. Education was segregated and impoverished for many of them. There were few books and reading was not encouraged. Thus, years of education (the biggest influence on BNT scores in the Ross, Lichtenberg, and Christensen, 1995 study), while a strong predictor of BNT scores, did not fully capture these cultural issues. It seems clear that exposure to the items on the BNT, primarily through reading, was different for whites and African Americans.

TABLE 5.11. Comparison of BNT Normative Data Between Optimally Healthy and Cognitively Intact Older Medical Patients

A. VanGorp et al. (1986). Community Sample (M = 37%, F = 63%)

Subjects' Age	Sample Size	Mean Years Education	Mean VIQ	Mean BNT
65 - 69 yrs	20	14.4 (2.3)*	123.0	55.6 (4.2)
70 - 74 yrs	24	15.2 (3.3)	130.0	54.4 (5.7)
75 - 79 yrs	13	14.2 (3.5)	115.0	51.6 (6.2)
80+ yrs	9	15.2 (4.5)	118.0	51.5 (7.0)

B. Mitrushina and Satz (1989). Community Sample (M = 39%, F = 61%)

Subjects' Age	Sample Size	Mean Years Education	Mean FSIQ	Mean BNT
66 - 70 yrs	45	14 (2.0)	119.3 (14.5)	55.8 (3.1)
71 - 75 yrs	57	14.6 (3.4)	118.7 (10.8)	53.0 (7.3)
76 - 85 yrs	26	13.3 (3.6)	112.0 (11.7)	50.8 (7.0)

C. Ross, Lichtenberg, and Christensen (1995). Medical Sample (M = 38%, F = 62%) (Black = 60%, White = 40%)

Subjects' Age	Sample Size	Mean Years Education	Mean DRS	Mean BNT
70 - 74 yrs	40	11.3 (3.1)	133.2 (4.48)	43.1 (11.7)
75 - 79 yrs	40	10.6 (3.3)	133.4 (4.75)	40.1 (10.9)
80+ yrs	43	10.2 (3.2)	131.4 (4.83)	35.8 (11.3)

Note: *Standard deviations are listed in parentheses.

TABLE 5.12. Item Listing of Boston Naming Test

Easy	BNT01+BNT02+BNT03+BNT04+BNT05+BNT06+BNT07+ BNT08+BNT09+BNT10+BNT11+BNT12+BNT14+BNT15+ BNT16+BNT17+BNT18+BNT20+BNT21+BNT28.
Moderate	BNT13+BNT19+BNT22+BNT23+BNT25+BNT26+BNT27+ BNT30+BNT31+BNT32+BNT33+BNT34+BNT35+BNT36+ BNT37+BNT38+BNT40+BNT46+BNT47+BNT49.
Hard	BNT24+BNT29+BNT39+BNT41+BNT42+BNT43+BNT44+ BNT45+BNT48+BNT50+BNT51+BNT52+BNT53+BNT54+ BNT55+BNT56+BNT57+BNT58+BNT59+BNT60.

To address the issue of clinical utility, we compared BNT scores from the 123 cognitively intact patients with the scores of 151 cognitively impaired patients. The cognitively impaired group was comparable to the cognitively intact group in terms of race and sex of the patients. The impaired group did, however, have a higher mean age (M = 80, SD = 8) and a lower level of education (M = 9, SD = 3.6) than did the cognitively intact group. A Discriminant Function Analysis was used to predict cognitive status based on demographic information and BNT scores. Overall, 73 percent of cases were correctly classified, with a sensitivity of .63 and a specificity of .80. In a follow-up study, 50 cognitively intact patients were compared with 50 cognitively impaired patients, this time matching the patients on age and education (Lichtenberg et al., in press). The results were identical to the findings described above. Thus, the BNT does not demonstrate the high rate of specificity that we found with the DRS, Logical Memory I and II, and the Fuld Object Memory Evaluation.

VISUOSPATIAL ABILITIES: VISUAL FORM DISCRIMINATION TEST

The Visual Form Discrimination Test (VFD) developed by Benton, Hamsher, Varney and Spreen (1983) is an appealing instrument to use with medically ill elderly because of its administration format. First, it is a nonmotoric task and can be used with patients suffering from hemiparesis or severe arthritis of the hands. Second, administration of the VFD is relatively brief. Empirical work on the VFD is quite limited. In their normative description of the VFD, Benton and colleagues (1983) included 27 subjects aged 55 to 75 years old. They found no difference on VFD scores between this group and the younger group (n = 58; ages 16 to 54) used in the normative sample. A second sample of 58 neurologically impaired patients (ages 16 to 68) were then used to determine the sensitivity of the VFD. The greatest sensitivity (71 percent correct classification) was found with the group suffering from bilateral and diffuse cerebral dysfunction. Because progressive dementias in the elderly often present with diffuse symptoms of cerebral dysfunction, the VFD may be a useful instrument to include in screening exams for dementia.

Moses (1986, 1989) studied the factor structure of many of Benton's tests (including the VFD) to determine if they provided information that was different from verbal learning and memory tasks. In the first set of studies, he used 97 middle-aged patients (M = 50; SD = 15) with neurologic and psychiatric diagnoses. Moses concluded that the VFD involved more active, perceptual processing than did simple copying tasks on the Benton Visual Retention Test. In addition, he noted that the VFD was differentiated from the Rey Auditory Verbal Learning Test (AVLT) scores as evidenced by its loading on a different factor than the AVLT. In Moses' second set of factor analytic studies, he increased his sample size to 162. The findings were essentially the same as in the first set of studies. The VFD thus appears to measure a different cognitive process than do tests of verbal learning and memory. Taken together, the results described above suggest that the VFD may be a useful test in screening for dementia. The VFD is sensitive to diffuse cerebral dysfunction and measures different cognitive processes than do tests of verbal learning and memory. Thus, we added the VFD to the test battery and undertook two studies to examine its normative properties and its clinical utility with our patients.

The initial normative data were produced on 30 patients with a mean age of 74 years (SD = 6.9) and a mean education of 10.5 years (SD = 3.2; Lichtenberg, Millis, and Nanna, 1994). In this sample, demographic variables (age, sex, education, race) were unrelated to VFD scores. As can be seen in Table 5.13, the mean scores in our sample were significantly lower than those reported by Benton et al. (1983). The normative study of the VFD was replicated in a larger sample (Nabors, Vangel, and Lichtenberg, in press).

The clinical utility of the VFD was examined first by Lichtenberg, Millis, and Nanna (1994), and replicated by Nabors, Vangel, and Lichtenberg (in press). In the Lichtenberg study, the cognitively impaired group was comprised of 31 patients. This group was significantly older than the intact patients (M = 79 years, SD = 7.2 years), but there was no difference between the groups in terms of education, sex, and race. Cutting scores were calculated to optimize sensitivity and specificity. At a cutting score of 23, there was 90 percent specificity and 67 percent sensitivity.

TABLE 5.13. Normative Observations for Older Adults on the Visual Form Discrimination Test

Author	Age	Education	VFD Score
Benton et al. (1983)	55 - 75	12	29.3
Lichtenberg et al. (in press)	74.1 (7)*	10.5 (3)	25.8 (3)
Sample Sizes			
Benton et al. (n = 25)			
Lichtenberg et al. (n = 31)			

Note: *Standard deviations are listed in parentheses.

Nabors, Vangel, and Lichtenberg (in press) increased the sample size to 184 subjects, with 92 comprising the cognitively unimpaired group, and 92 comprising the cognitively impaired group. In the cognitively unimpaired group, VFD scores were significantly correlated with education (r = .19, p<.05) and race (r = .24, p<.05), such that white patients having a higher level of education tended to obtain higher VFD scores. Overall, demographic variables accounted for 10 percent of VFD variance in the cognitively unimpaired group.

The cognitively unimpaired group was significantly younger (mean age of 75 years versus 76 years) and more educated (mean years of education of 11 years versus 9 years). The groups did not differ with respect to race and to gender. Similar to the Lichtenberg, Ross, and Christenson study (1994), the cognitively intact group had a mean VFD score of 25 (SD = 4.5), whereas the impaired group had a mean VFD score of 19.8 (SD = 5.3). Logistic regression analysis was used to determine the extent to which cases could be correctly assigned based on VFD scores and relevant demographic information. When age, race, and education were entered, the correct classification was 66 percent overall, with 67 percent specificity and 64 percent sensitivity. With the addition of VFD scores, correct classification increased to 73 percent overall, with a specificity of 75 percent and a sensitivity of 72 percent. Only age and VFD scores were significant predictors in this equation. Cutting scores were then calculated for the VFD. As with the previous research, a cut score of 23 resulted in the highest correct classification overall, with a specificity of 68 percent and a sensitivity at 73 percent.

HOOPER VISUAL ORGANIZATION TEST

The Hooper Visual Organization Test (VOT) (Hooper, 1958) was initially developed to discriminate brain damaged from non–brain-damaged psychiatric patients. Love's (1970) data provided support for the validity of the VOT. He compared VOT scores for 20 psychiatric patients with known organic conditions to 95 psychiatric patients thought not to have neurologic involvement. Using a cutoff score of 20, he reported a sensitivity of .70 and a specificity of .86. Gerson (1974) compared 16 patients with organic brain damage to 19 psychiatric patients thought not to have organic involvement, and to 33 cognitively intact, non-psychiatrically impaired individuals. He matched these groups for age and IQ. He concluded that the VOT was useful in identifying brain-damaged individuals, but was not useful in discriminating between psychiatric patients without brain damage and normal controls. Boyd (1981) also found that a group of psychiatric patients without known organic brain damage scored significantly higher on the VOT than did a group of brain damaged controls.

Normative data for the VOT has been limited for older adults. While Hooper's (1958) norms do account for age and education, they do not extend past age 69. Montgomery and Costa (1983) reported a mean score of 22.5 (SD = 4.1) for a group of 82 healthy adults aged 65 to 89, but did not report level of education. In a recent study of healthy community older adult volunteers, a clear difference was found between a young-old and an old-old group (Libon et al., 1994). In this study, the young-old group (M = 70 years) had a mean VOT score of 23.1 (SD = 4), whereas the old-old group (M = 81 years) had a mean VOT score of 19.9 (SD = 3). Educational levels for both groups had a mean greater than 12 years. Normative data on the VOT is, thus, clearly lacking for less educated older adults, and no norms have been generated for African Americans on the VOT.

Nabors and colleagues (in press) collected VOT data from 58 cognitively intact and 59 cognitively impaired older adult patients.

The cognitively intact group was 75 percent female, 57 percent African American, and had a mean level of education of 11 years (SD = 3.2) and a mean age of 76 years (SD = 6.1). The cognitively impaired group was significantly older (M = 79, SD = 6.6) and less educated (M = 8.8, SD = 3.4) than was the intact group. Sixty percent of the impaired group were women and 50 percent were African American. The difference between the groups in terms of racial composition was not significant.

Correlational analyses for the cognitively intact group revealed that VOT scores were unrelated to age (r = -.05), race (r = -.01), gender (r = .01), and education (r = .06). This lack of relationship was surprising given the findings of Libon and colleagues. While a larger sample may be needed to obtain a more valid indication of the relationship between demographic variables and VOT scores, an alternative explanation is proposed here. As can be seen in Table 5.14, the mean scores for the cognitively intact group are lower than Libon et al.'s groups, and even are below Hooper's cutoff scores. It may be that due to some of the ease of the early test items and the difficulty on the later test items there is a raised floor effect, and a low ceiling effect, thereby restricting the range of scores (see Table 5.14).

The clinical utility of the VOT was assessed through a Discriminant Function Analysis and through cutoff scores. The mean VOT score for the impaired group was 11.4 (SD = 4.4). The VOT was able to classify 79 percent of the cases overall, with an 80 percent specificity and a 78 percent sensitivity. A cutoff score of 15 provided the best classification overall (81 percent sensitivity, 79 percent specificity). These results point to the validity of utilizing the VOT with our elderly patient population. The relatively low specificity should remind clinicians to be cautious in their VOT score interpretations and not use the VOT as their only screening measure.

THE NSRP TEST BATTERY

The NSRP test battery consists of all the tests reviewed above and several other tests that have yet to be adequately researched (see Table 5.15). The test battery takes between 75 minutes to two hours. As can be seen in the table, memory testing is emphasized.

TABLE 5.14. Normative Observations for Older Adults on the Hooper Visual Organization Test

Author	Age	Education	VOT Score
Montgomery and Costa (1983)	65 to 89	unknown	22.5 (4)*
Libon et al. (1994)	69.7 (3)	13.4 (3)	23.1 (4)
Libon et al. (1994)	81.0 (4)	12.4 (3)	19.9 (3)
Walsh, Lichtenberg, and Rowe (1997)	73.2	11.7 (3)	18.6 (5)

Sample Sizes

Montgomery and Costa (n = 82)

Libon et al. (young-old n = 23)

         (old-old n = 14)

Walsh and Lichtenberg (n = 32)

Note: *Standard deviations are listed in parentheses.

Tests that tap into the domains of language, visuospatial skills, and executive functioning are also included, as is a test of reading.

Determining which reading test to use posed some challenges to the NSRP test battery. Reading has been shown in cross-sectional and longitudinal studies to decline, during a dementia, at a slower rate than other cognitive abilities (Ryan and Paolo, 1992; Paque and Warrington, 1995). Reading can thus be used to estimate premorbid levels of intellectual functioning. We initially chose to use the National Adult Reading Test-Revised (NART-R) (Blair and Spreen, 1989), but switched to the large print form of the Wide Range Achievement Test–Revised (WRAT-R). Scores on the NART-R were consistently poor, and in keeping with the findings of Wiens, Bryan, Crossen (1993), the WRAT-R provided better discrimination of scores at the lower levels of intellectual functioning. Other findings gave us confidence about the WRAT-R, such as consistent correlations between WRAT-R and education for both whites ($r = .67$ $p<.05$) and African Americans ($r = .68$, $p<.05$).

TABLE 5.15. NRSP Test Battery

- WRAT-R Reading
- Multilingual Aphasia Examination (MAE) Aural Comprehension
- Mattis Dementia Rating Scale
- Logical Memory Subtests
- Boston Naming Test
- Visual Form Discrimination Test
- Hooper Visual Organization Test
- Fuld Object Memory Exam
- Verbal Fluency (CFL and Animals)
- Geriatric Depression Scale
- CAGE Questions for Alcohol Abuse

FACTOR ANALYSIS OF THE NSRP TEST BATTERY

A factor analysis was conducted on a sample of 237 patients who received the following tests: Dementia Rating Scale, Boston Naming Test, Hooper Visual Organization Test, Visual Form Discrimination Test, and Logical Memory I and II. Of the 247 patients, 74 were cognitively intact and fully independent in ADL abilities, 89 were cognitively impaired and had deficiencies in at least three ADLs, and the remaining 73 patients were either cognitively intact but had ADL deficiencies or cognitively impaired but had few ADL limitations. The mean scores for the cognitive tests and the demographic measures can be found in Table 5.16. As can be seen in the table, the mean age was in the late 70s, mean education was 10.4 years, 68 percent of the sample were women, and 56 percent of the sample were African Americans.

Intercorrelations among the measures can be found in Table 5.17. As can be seen in the table all correlations were significant beyond the .001 level, ranging from a low of $r = .32$ between Logical Memory I (WMS-R Immediate) and Visual Form Discrimination Test to a high of $r = .81$ between Logical Memory I and Logical Mmemory II. That the Hooper Visual Organization Test and the

TABLE 5.16. Descriptive Statistics for 237 Patients with Complete NSRP Battery Data

	Mean	Standard Deviation	Range	n (%)
NSRP BATTERY (n = 237)				
Boston Naming Test	37.79	13.69	12 - 60	n.a.
Dementia Rating Scale	121.15	14.89	71 - 143	n.a.
Hooper VOT	15.30	5.42	3 - 30	n.a.
Visual Form	22.40	5.62	0 - 32	n.a.
WMS-R Immediate	15.11	6.86	0 - 33	n.a.
WMS-R Delayed	10.79	6.67	0 - 28	n.a.
WRAT-R READING (n = 190)	48.43	17.79	0 - 87	n.a.
COMORBIDITY INDEX (n = 178)	1.85	1.40	0 - 7	n.a.
DEMOGRAPHICS (n = 237)				
Age	77.46	6.37	61 - 94	n.a.
Education (Years)	10.38	3.51	0 - 20	n.a.
Gender: Male	n.a.	n.a.	n.a.	75 (32%)
Female	n.a.	n.a.	n.a.	162 (68%)
Race: African-American	n.a.	n.a.	n.a.	134 (56%)
White	n.a.	n.a.	n.a.	103 (44%)
IMPAIRMENT RATING (n = 163)				
Intact	n.a.	n.a.	n.a.	74 (45%)
Impaired	n.a.	n.a.	n.a.	89 (55%)

TABLE 5.17. Intercorrelation of NSRP Battery Measures (n = 237)

	1	2	3	4	5	6
1. Boston Naming Test	—					
2. Dementia Rating Scale	.59	—				
3. Hooper VOT	.63	.55	—			
4. Visual Form	.53	.61	.53	—		
5. WMS-R Immediate	.53	.49	.37	.32	—	
6. WMS-R Delayed	.52	.56	.40	.36	.81	—

Note: All correlations in the above table are significant at $p < .001$.

Visual Form Discrimination Test were so highly correlated with measures of language, verbal memory and general cognitive functioning was surprising.

A Principal Components Analysis was conducted in order to determine how many factors the NSRP test battery was measuring. As can be seen in Table 5.18, 60 percent of the variance was explained overall and there was only one factor derived. Loadings were very consistent and high, ranging from .71 to .82. These findings are drastically different from both those of the CERAD battery, which found three factors, and the findings of Moses (1986, 1989), in which verbal memory and visuospatial abilities loaded on separate factors. Our interpretation of this finding is that in this urban population with a majority of less educated and African-American patients, the tests are all measuring the same construct, cognition. This finding was quite unexpected, but underlined the need for developing test batteries and conducting research on psychometric properties on urban African-American and white samples. As will be seen later in the chapter, without exception, the means and standard deviations for these tests with our urban samples were lower than norms published on optimally healthy, highly educated white community samples. Level of difficulty thus may be responsible for the high relationship among all tests, and for a lack of different strengths or weaknesses (e.g., verbal memory versus visuospatial measures).

TABLE 5.18. Principal Components Analysis of NSRP Battery (n = 237)

	Loading
Boston Naming Test	.82
Dementia Rating Scale	.82
Hooper VOT	.75
Visual Form	.76
WMS-R Immediate	.79
WMS-R Delayed	.71
Eigenvalue	3.61
Percent Variance Explained	60.2%

Logistic regression analysis was performed to determine the clinical utility of the test battery in classifying cognitively unimpaired patients from mildly impaired patients. Due to the one factor solution described above, and the high multicolinearity among variables, the four variables with the lowest intercorrelations were entered into the regression: Dementia Rating Scale (DRS), Logical Memory I (LMI), Visual Form Discrimination (VFD), and Hooper Visual Organization Test (VOT). A forward forced-entry selection was utilized here so as to parallel the findings from the Christensen, Paulovic-Hadzi, and Jacomb (1991) meta-analytic study. The DRS was entered first as a measure of general cognition. The DRS was a significant predictor of intact and impaired cases (Chi Square = 36.03, p<.01), with an overall accurate classification of 75 percent. Sensitivity was at 77 percent, and specificity was at 74 percent. The DRS had a positive predictive power of 72 percent and a negative predictive power of 79 percent; that is, the DRS was relatively better at classifying cognitively unimpaired patients than it was in classifying cognitively impaired patients. The addition of the other tests (memory, then visuospatial, then language) did not improve the logistic regression. This finding is consistent with the finding of one factor. Overall then, the regression analysis demonstrated that the DRS improved classification of unimpaired versus impaired cases well over population base rates, but also had a relatively high rate of false positives (33 percent).

Clinical Implications of the NSRP Battery

The data clearly indicate the usefulness of the NSRP test battery for older adult urban medical patients. There was relatively good discrimination between cognitively unimpaired and impaired older urban medical patients. There were unique findings, however, regarding the neuropsychological profiles of our samples as compared to those reported with previous samples. All of the tests loaded on a single factor, and improved incremental validity was not found by adding tests to a regression equation. Means and standard deviations were lower, overall, on all NSRP tests except the Fuld and the Dementia Rating Scale. African Americans scored significantly lower on the Boston Naming Test and the Visual Form Discrimination Test, as compared to whites. Race as a variable, however, explains nothing. It is used merely as a crude index of cultural differences. While it is clear that cultural influences have a great influence on neuropsychological test results, it is not at all clear how to best measure the effects of culture. Thus, we are left with age, education, sex, race, income, and occupational status as crude markers of cultural background.

Some test scores were influenced more by demographic variables than were others in our sample. The Dementia Rating Scale and the Fuld Object Memory Evaluation had norms identical to those established on white samples having a higher level of education than our sample. The Logical Memory subtests, the Hooper Visual Organization Test, and the Visual Form Discrimination Test were only modestly related to demographic variables in our sample, but displayed significantly lower mean scores than those reported in previous normative studies using white subjects who were more highly educated than our sample. The Boston Naming Test was particularly influenced by demographic variables and had lower means than previously published norms. Thus, while we advocate for the usage of the NSRP test battery, we implore all to interpret scores cautiously.

Chapter 6

Utilizing the NSRP Test Battery

CASE ILLUSTRATIONS WITH THE NSRP TEST BATTERY

The following cases are presented here to provide some clinical illustrations regarding the types of diagnostic and practical information that can be gleaned through the NSRP test battery. Each case vignette will contain a brief history, test scores, a discussion of diagnosis, and applications to everyday functioning. It is imperative to remember that neuropsychological test scores alone are not sufficient to diagnose dementia. Rather, the essential process is to incorporate test scores with a patient's history. One way to utilize the case studies is to first omit the history and conclusion sections, and to look only at the test data. Match the patient's age and education to the normative data available. Then utilize three questions to guide your interpretation of test data: (1) Is there evidence of cognitive deficits? (2) What are the cognitive strengths and weaknesses? and (3) What practical recommendations can you make? After you have done this, then go back and review the history and conclusions and compare your answers with ours. While this section will apply most directly to psychologists who work in health care settings, mental health practitioners from all disciplines can benefit from exposure to how psychological test results can be applied to actual cases.

CASE #1: MRS. M

Mrs. M was an 81-year-old, white, widowed, retired secretary who entered the hospital after falling and laying on the floor for two days until she was discovered by her niece. After one week in the general hospital, she came to the geriatric rehabilitation unit. Mrs. M's other medical problems included hypertension, aortic stenosis, and a mild arrhythmia. She had completed ten years of education. During her rehabilitation stay she was given the NSRP test battery, and two months subsequent to her discharge from the rehabilitation unit, she was given a second neuropsychological evaluation. Scores are provided below.

	Testing #1	Testing #2
Dementia Rating Scale	114	123
Attention	36	36
Initiation/Perseveration	19	26
Construction	3	4
Conceptualization	34	33
Memory	22	24
WRAT-R Reading (scaled score)	94	95
Logical Memory I	16	19
Logical Memory II	4	14
Fuld Storage	36	43
Fuld Retrieval	30	35
Fuld Repeated Retrieval	17	23
Fuld Ineffective Reminders	8	5
VFD	29	30
VOT	13	17
BNT	36	45
GDS	8	5

Is there evidence of cerebral dysfunction?

On Testing #1, Mrs. M's reading score was used to estimate her premorbid level of intellectual functioning to have been in the average range, consistent with her years of education. Test results represented a decline in cognitive functioning than what would be expected based on normative data.

What are her cognitive strengths and weaknesses?

Specifically, Mrs. M displayed mild cognitive impairment overall on the DRS, with a relative weakness noted in simple copying, and in word generation. Memory tests indicated significant problems with encoding and retrieval. Although her score on Logical Memory I was in the unimpaired range, on Logical Memory II she only recalled 25 percent of what was originally remembered. On the Fuld there were indications of impaired learning, although retrieval indices on the Fuld did not appear impaired. Finally, whereas Mrs. M's score on a task of matching designs was unimpaired (VFD), her score was in the moderately impaired range for a more complex visuospatial task (VOT).

What practical recommendations can be made?

The results of this evaluation were used to recommend that Mrs. M not return to living alone at this time. Due to her memory problems, it was thought she would be unable to correctly take her own medications, to prepare meals consistently, and to pay her bills. She was discharged to her niece's home.

Mrs. M returned for a follow-up evaluation at her request because she believed that her mind was clearing up, and that her memory had returned to unimpaired functioning. The test scores indicated significant improvements in cognitive functioning. Mrs. M's DRS score increased by 9 points, or 1 1/2 standard deviations. Memory functioning, as measured by Logical Memory and the Fuld, was significantly improved as well. To guard against practice effects, the California Verbal Learning Test was also given, and Mrs. M scored in the unimpaired range on all indices. Her problem-solving skills improved, as evidenced by her increased VOT scores. Her niece reported that Mrs. M had been gardening, performing all of her own ADLs, and was accurately using a pillbox system to dispense medications. These results indicated that Mrs. M was cognitively capable of returning to living alone. She and her niece devised a daily check-in system, and Mrs. M returned home.

This case is presented first to underscore the following: Diagnoses of a progressive dementia should not be made on the basis of a single episode of impaired test scores. Lichtenberg (1994) highlighted the need for longitudinal evaluations. This was underscored, recently, by a longitudinal study of "cognitively impaired normal elderly" who, although they scored in the impaired range on initial testing, displayed no further cognitive decline after three to five years (Malec et al.,

1996). It is particularly true that caution be used in interpreting test scores for hospitalized elderly. In the case of Mrs. M deconditioning, dehydration and weakness were likely causes of her cognitive decline due to their generalized effects on cognitive performance and brain efficiency. These effects were reversible. For other elderly, improved glycemic or hypertensive control may produce improved cognitive functioning in older adults suffering from diabetes or hypertension (Meneilly et al., 1993; Salerno et al., 1995).

CASE #2: MS. MF

Ms. MF was a 75-year-old, African-American, widowed, retired schoolteacher who had a left hip replacement due to long-term degenerative joint disease. Other medical problems included hypertension and hypothyroidism. For the past four years, she used a cane at home to ambulate, but Ms. MF was independent in all of her ADLs and IADLs, including cooking. She retired 14 years prior to her surgery, and had enjoyed the freedom of retirement and traveling. Ms. MF was referred for an evaluation because she lived alone. She had completed 18 years of education.

Dementia Rating Scale (total) 143
Logical Memory I 28
Logical Memory II 24
BNT 58
VFD 32
VOT 25
WRAT-R (scaled score) 110
GDS 0

Is there evidence of cerebral impairment?

Ms. MF's case is an example of successful aging. There are no test scores indicative of any cognitive decline. We put this case in to drive home the point that many practitioners do not get the chance to be exposed to cognitively intact older adults. For practitioners it can be detrimental to not have observed normal and successful aging. Exposure to old adults is invaluable, if for no other reason than to curb any ageist attitudes or biases.

CASE #3: MS. P

Ms. P was a 79-year-old, African-American, widowed, retired beauty shop operator whose knee pain worsened over several years to the point of being unable to ambulate. Ms. P was admitted for a right knee replacement. Other medical problems included anemia. Prior to her rehabilitation admission, Ms. P received Meals on Wheels, had friends who performed most of her IADLs, but did take care of her own ADLs. Ms. P did continue to drive on occasion. She completed 13 years of school. Her friend of 50 years described to me that Ms. P was often becoming confused, with decreased memory and concentration. A neuropsychological evaluation was conducted.

Dementia Rating Scale 114
Attention 35
Initiation/Perseveration 21
Construction 6
Conceptualization 37
Memory 15
Logical Memory I 6
Logical memory II 0
Fuld Storage 20
Fuld Retrieval 11
Fuld Repeated Retrieval 4
Ineffective Reminders 26
BNT 24
WRAT-R Reading (scaled score) 88
MAE Aural Comprehension 17
VFD 30
VOT 15

Is there evidence of cerebral dysfunction?

Ms. P's test results are consistent with a primary progressive dementia such as Alzheimer's disease. While her reading score indicates premorbid cognitive functioning levels to have been in the average range, her scores on other tests, particularly tests of memory and naming, are significantly impaired.

What are her cognitive strengths and weaknesses?

Indeed the test results indicate that attentional skills can be relatively well preserved in early dementia, as evidenced by her score on the VFD. Aural comprehension is unimpaired, but confrontation naming is reduced. Scores on both memory tests are severely reduced, with the Fuld scores being some of the lowest scores that we have seen.

What practical recommendations can be made?

Due to the severity of Ms. P's memory problems, it was recommended that she receive 24-hour supervision. Her dear friend took Ms. P into her home, but after six months, Ms. P had declined further (she was seen after a fall brought her back into the rehabilitation unit) and was transferred to a nursing home. In the interim period, she had received a thorough work-up to rule out reversible causes of her cognitive decline, and been diagnosed with probable Alzheimer's disease.

CASE #4: MRS. V

The following patient was referred to me by a defense attorney for an auto insurance company. The patient was complaining of cognitive problems subsequent to a head injury three years prior to my evaluation. Below is a brief description of her accident, and the test results.

A 72-year-old, white, married homemaker underwent a neuropsychological evaluation to determine whether she experienced brain injury from a motor vehicle accident and to determine whether this brain injury was disabling to her at the time of the evaluation. Mrs. V reported that she was a restrained passenger when she and her husband were rear-ended by a vehicle traveling at approximately 40 miles per hour and then were broadsided by this same vehicle moments later. According to the hospital records, the patient denied head or neck injury at the time, but complained of lower back and leg pain. According to the patient, she did not lose consciousness, but became confused immediately after the accident, and she said she has become increasingly confused since then. According to neurology notes from one year after the accident, she underwent an EEG, which showed some slowing in the right hemisphere compatible with vascular problems. She underwent a neuropsychological evaluation two years after the accident, in which it was concluded that there was diffuse cerebral dysfunction, primarily in the left hemisphere. My testing was completed one year after her first neuropsychological evaluation. She had completed eight years of education and was a homemaker her entire adult life.

Prior to initiating the neuropsychological evaluation, I informed the patient about the purpose of this evaluation, about the limits of confidentiality with regard to the evaluation, and I cautioned her to give her best effort, and not to intentionally perform poorly. She told me that she would try her best.

Zarit Self-Memory Assessment: 50 percent loss of memory estimated

WRAT-R Reading (scaled score) 79

Dementia Rating Scale 109

Attention 35

Initiation 20

Construction 6

Conceptualization 35

Memory 13 (including 3/9 on recognition tasks)

MAE Comprehension 17

Boston Naming Test 20

Visual Form discrimination 20

Hooper Visual Organization Test 13

Controlled Oral Word Association (COWAT) 15

Animal Naming 3

Fuld Storage 27

   Retrieval 19

   Repeated Retrieval 9

   Ineffective Reminders 19

Warrington Recognition Memory Test 26/50 (- 5+ s.d.); 16 correct of 1st 25; then missed last 8 responses in last 25.

Logical Memory I and II begun but not given because patient informed examiner that she had these tests in the last testing.

Geriatric Depression Scale 23

*Inconsistencies Between Patient's Report
and That of Her Husband and Friend*

On a self-report memory measure, Mrs. V rated her memory as severely impaired, and much worse than others her age. Despite this, Mrs. V was able to chronicle the multitude of medical problems she has experienced since the accident. Upon interview, her husband stated that he did not notice any problems with his wife's memory. Her friend also confided that Mrs. V's memory appeared to be working well to him. On a test of verbal recognition memory Mrs. V scored at the level of chance. This pattern of results is consistent with someone who is experiencing a moderate to severe progressive dementia, or alternately, the pattern of her performance on this test raises suspicion that she was motivated to answer questions incorrectly. On a test of selective reminding, Mrs. V's score was in the severely impaired range. Again, the level of performance and pattern of performance on this test both raise suspicion about the truthfulness of her responses.

Mrs. V reported symptoms of severe depression and symptoms of severe post-traumatic stress disorder. She stated that she ruminates about the accident, will very rarely allow herself to be in a car, is frightened often, dreams about the car wreck frequently, and has a sense of impending doom. She also claimed to have a severe sleep onset and early waking problem. According to her husband, Mrs. V's sleeping has not deteriorated since before the accident, nor has he noted symptoms of fear or depression—"only physical pain." What is consistent among Mrs. V and the other two informants is that she was an extremely busy and active woman prior to the accident and is no longer active at all.

Is there evidence of cerebral impairment?

The pattern of results with which Mrs. V presented led to differentiating between a primary progressive dementia in the moderate to severely impaired stage or a conscious or unconscious attempt to make herself appear brain damaged. The severity of her impaired scores on memory and language tasks would fall in the range of someone experiencing moderate to severe dementia. Based upon her medical records, and her husband's and friends' reports, however, it is known that Mrs. V suffered from a mild head injury. Her performance of independent ADLs and IADLs is inconsistent with a severe dementia. Her profile, therefore, is not consistent: Her test scores are more severe than would be expected based upon her functional skills and the injury she suffered. In a series of papers, Millis (1992, 1994) provided data validating the use of the Warrington Recognition Memory test (RMT) in the detection of exaggerated responding or malingering. In Mrs. V's case, her RMT score was at chance level, indicating that absolutely no learning had occurred. This score was well below the cutoff scores provided by Millis.

What practical recommendations can be made?

By considering the combination of a self-reported history of cognitive and emotional problems that was not supported by her husband or her friend, along with a pattern of test results consistent with exaggerated performance, the following conclusion was reached. "This neuropsychological evaluation found no evidence of brain dysfunction. What was clear, however, was that Mrs. V responded in a way that would make her appear to have severe cognitive and emotional problems."

CASE #5: MR. W

Mr. W was a 76-year-old retired factory worker who entered the hospital for chest pain three weeks prior to his neuropsychological evaluation. He suffered a heart attack. Other medical problems include hypertension, non–insulin-dependent diabetes mellitus, and a coronary bypass surgery three years previously. Before this hospitalization, Mr. W was living with his wife. He was independent with all of his ADLs and was driving. He completed 12 years of education. His test scores follow.

WRAT-R Reading (scaled score) 85
DRS Total 118
Attention 36
Initiation/Perseveration 30
Construction 5

Conceptualization 34
Memory 13
MAE Aural Comprehension 18
Boston Naming Test 37
Logical Memory I 11
Logical Memory II 0
Fuld Storage 26
Fuld Retrieval 18
Fuld Repeated Retrieval 9
Fuld Ineffective Reminders 20
Visual Form Discrimination 21
Hooper VOT 18.5
Controlled Oral Word 20
Geriatric Depression Scale 2

Is there evidence of cognitive impairment?

In the case of Mr. W, comparison of his scores to normative data reveals that on all indices of memory (Logical Memory and the Fuld) he scored significantly below the normative data. In the Logical Memory II subtest, for example, his percent retained was 0, and in the Fuld Storage he scored several standard deviations below the mean. These low scores on memory tests are in sharp contrast to his reading score, which was in the average range.

What are the cognitive strengths and weaknesses?

Mr. W displays many strengths, particularly in the areas of language (including naming), visuoperceptual, and visuo-organizational skills. Weaknesses are notable in both memory and mental flexibility tasks. At this point, it is useful to integrate the findings with the history so as to be able to help with diagnostic issues. The onset of Mr. W's cognitive deficits was rather sudden, occurring immediately after the apparent heart attack. Thus, these results are not likely due to previously existing progressive dementia. The pattern of results, linked with the history of a heart attack and sudden onset of severe memory dysfunction, are also entirely consistent with a hypoxic episode. In hypoxic episodes, the hippocampal regions are particularly susceptible to damage (Albert and Knoefel, 1994), correlating with the severe memory deficits seen here.

What practical recommendations can be made?

The test results have profound implications for Mr. W's lifestyle. Given his cognitive deficits, he may not be able to drive, manage his own medications, cook without supervision, or manage household finances. Assessment of these skills in his occupational therapies proved that he needed help in all the tasks mentioned above. Mrs. W will have to assume the role of 24-hour caregiver. It was also recommended that Mrs. W petition the court for guardianship.

CASE #6: MS. P

Ms. P was an 82-year-old married woman who acted as a caregiver to her 97-year-old husband. She fell and broke her hip, forcing her to undergo surgery and physical rehabilitation. Other medical problems included a history of non–insulin-dependent diabetes mellitus, hypertension, transient ischemic events (stroke symptoms that had sudden onset, and then resolved within one day), and obesity. Ms. P was referred for an evaluation because she was barely making any progress in her physical therapies. She was seen on two occasions, separated by a two-week interval. At the first interview, Ms. P was lethargic and barely able to attend to our questions. The nurses reported that Ms. P was not sleeping well, was emotionally labile at times, and appeared frightened.

	Time 1	Time 2
Dementia Rating Scale (total)	87	99
Attention	32	32
Initiation/Perseveration	23	25
Construction	3	4
Conceptualization	20	21
Memory	9	17
Fuld Storage	20	29
Fuld Retrieval	10	15

Fuld Repeated Retrieval	4	7
Fuld Ineffective Reminders	29	23
Visual Form Discrimination	12	17

Is there evidence of cerebral impairment?

The behavioral presentation of Ms. P at Time 1 is consistent with a delirium. A delirium is a transient or subacute encephalopathy caused by any number of medical or drug conditions. A thorough review of delirium is presented by LaRue (1993), and delirium assessment instruments can also be found (Albert et al., 1992; Trzepacz, Baker, and Greenhouse, 1987). Ms. P's delirium was caused by a urinary tract infection, one of the most common underlying causes of delirium in medically ill elderly (Rockwood, 1993).

What practical recommendations can be made?

A longitudinal approach to assessment can be used with delirious patients. The reversibility of cognitive and functional decline in a delirious patient can be quite variable—from total reversibility to almost no reversibility. Of importance is that even after Ms. P's delirium cleared, there remained evidence of significant cognitive deficits. This underscores the point that demented individuals are the most vulnerable to the onset of a delirium. After these test findings were noted with Ms. P, a more careful questioning of her daughter led to the apparent two- to three-year history of cognitive decline in Ms. P. These results had clear implications about her abilities to manage herself, let alone her husband. The family opted to provide 24-hour supervision to the couple.

CASE #7: MS. H

Ms. H was an 85-year-old, African-American, widowed, retired custodial worker who was admitted to the hospital after she collapsed while cleaning her apartment. She was then unable to stand or walk and was taken to the hospital by her sister. Prior to this episode of falling, Ms. H had been living alone in a senior citizen's apartment, was independent with ambulation and all of her ADLs, and was independent with all of her IADLs including cooking and volunteering in her church. She had completed eight years of education.

Ms. H was diagnosed with severe dehydration following her admission to the hospital. A head CT scan found evidence of diffuse atrophy, but there was no evidence of any acute changes to the brain. Other medical problems included peripheral neuropathy, arthritis, hypertension, and deconditioning. She was initially referred for a neuropsychological evaluation to help determine if she was cognitively capable of returning to live alone. She was given a second set of cognitive tests 10 days later when acute changes in cognition were noted, as well as lethargy and new onset incontinence. She was given a third cognitive testing three weeks following the second testing to assess for improvement.

	Testing 1	*Testing 2*	*Testing 3*
WRAT-R Reading (scaled score)	86	89	89
Dementia Rating Scale (total)	96	84	103
Attention	35	31	35
Initiation/Perseveration	20	19	22
Construction	3	2	4
Conceptualization	23	21	25
Memory	15	11	17
Logical Memory I	8	0	9
Logical Memory II	4	0	4
Boston Naming Test	14	0	16
Visual Form discrimination	0	0	0

Is there evidence of cerebral dysfunction?

Our review of results at the first testing, combined with the history and CT scan results, led us to conclude that a more complete examination was needed in order to rule out a primary dementia. Severe cognitive deficits in language, memory, and problem solving were consistent with diffuse atrophy noted on the CT scan. These results were not consistent, however, with reports of Ms. H leading a very independent and active lifestyle prior to her injury. Nevertheless early symptoms of dementia can be overlooked by family members, and an episode of dehydration may simply have exacerbated the symptoms. Ten days later, however, Ms. H exhibited new signs

of neurologic dysfunction. She became totally disoriented, inconti-
nent, and displayed an abrupt change in cognition. A delirium was
suspected, and we recommended a repeat head CT scan.

The head CT took place 25 days after the initial scan, and displayed a new finding: a right parietal subdural hematoma. Because
of atrophy in her brain, Ms. H, like most older adults, was at risk for
a subdural hematoma even with only minor trauma (Albert and
Knoefel, 1994). The fall led to Ms. H hitting her head, and the onset
of symptoms of the subdural hematoma was delayed.

What are the cognitive strengths and weaknesses?

A third evaluation was conducted by us three weeks after Ms. H
received a surgical evacuation of the subdural hematoma. As can be
seen in the test results, there was considerable improvement in Ms.
H's performance as compared to Time 2, but at best slight improvement as compared to Time 1. These improvements included improvement in general cognitive functioning.

What practical recommendations can be made?

Clearly, significant cognitive deficits remained. Ms. H returned to
live with her sister. She was not tested by us again, but at a six-month
physician visit, Ms. H's sister reported that Ms. H was doing well
physically but had not regained good cognitive functioning.

CASE #8: MS. A

Ms. A was a 68-year-old, single (never married), white, retired
secretary who entered the hospital due to progressive weakness and
falling over a period of a week. Prior to this admission she lived
with her brother and sister in a two-story home. Her brother did the
driving, and for the past year her sister was taking over more of the
cooking and cleaning—tasks they used to share equally. Ms. A
retired four years prior to this hospitalization and had been active in
church and socially until one year ago when she simply began to not
feel well. Her only other medical problem was hypertension. She
had completed 12 years of education.

WRAT-R Reading (scaled score) 65
Dementia Rating Scale (total) 113
Attention 35
Initiation/Perseveration 33
Construction 1
Conceptualization 27
Memory 17
MAE Aural Comprehension 12
Boston Naming Test 20
Logical Memory I 6
Logical Memory II 4
Fuld Storage 45
Fuld Retrieval 32
Fuld Repeated Retrieval 16
Fuld Ineffective Reminders 5
Visual Form Discrimination 16
Hooper Visual Organization Test 10
Controlled Oral Word Test 21
Geriatric Depression Scale 4

Is there evidence of cerebral dysfunction?

This test protocol contains both classic features of a subcortical form of dementia and some features rarely seen in a dementia that emanates primarily due to subcortical lesions.

What are cognitive strengths and weaknesses?

To summarize briefly, Cummings (1993) describes the hallmark features of subcortical dementia as slowed information processing, retrieval deficits, and mental flexibility deficits, whereas language is typically found to be intact. Ms. A demonstrated extremely slowed information processing, requiring twice the amount of time than is usually required to complete testing. In addition, results from her Fuld indicate no problems encoding information but clear retrieval deficits. Finally, test results from the Hooper VOT and the Controlled Oral Word test indicate mental flexibility deficits. Other parts of the test results do not fit so neatly with classic subcortical dementia.

Inspection of Ms. A's reading, comprehension, naming and Logical Memory test scores indicate that she has significant aphasic difficulties. Her reading is well below that of a secretary, with a score in the defective range. Ms. A demonstrated severe problems with comprehension for basic information. Her score on the Boston Naming test also indicates some problems with word finding. Finally, it is interesting to see the impact of her aphasia on her ability to recall information that is verbal contextual (i.e., stories), whereas recall of items encoded through multiple means (touch, naming, seeing) are readily encoded on the Fuld. Following this evaluation, an MRI scan was obtained, and the results indicated a predominance of multifocal, deep white matter disease and some cortical atrophy.

What practical recommendations can be made?

Ms. A clearly was in need of more family support than she was receiving. Her communication difficulties made her attempts at some IADL activities (finances, shopping) ineffective. Her family was educated as to the usage of short, simple phrasing to communicate with Ms. A.

CASE #9: MS. H

Ms. H was a 74-year-old, white, married, retired beautician who entered our hospital two years after beginning to suffer from chronic back pain and three months after a laminectomy. She was noted to have severe back and hip problems and had undergone a hip replacement ten days prior to her admission for medical rehabilitation. Prior to her surgery, her pain was not well controlled and she was not walking the last six months. Other medical problems included nicotine addiction, diabetes mellitus, and hypertension. She was retired for ten years and had completed 14 years of education. She was referred for a cognitive evaluation because she "appeared somewhat demented" upon admission.

On the NSRP test battery for dementia, the following scores were obtained:

WRAT-R Reading (scaled score) 87
Dementia Rating Scale (total) 136
Attention 36
Initiation/Perseveration 35
Construction 6
Conceptualization 36
Memory 23
Logical Memory I 8
Logical Memory II 6
Boston Naming Test 32
Fuld Storage 45
Fuld Retrieval 39
Fuld Repeated Retrieval 23
Fuld Ineffective Reminders 2
Visual Form Discrimination 23
Hooper VOT 14
Controlled Oral Word 22

Is there evidence of cerebral impairment?

Ms. H's profile is consistent with subclinical impairments due to alcohol abuse (Ryan and Butters, 1986). Indeed, Ms. H's score on the CAGE questionnaire (a screening measure for alcohol abuse reviewed in a later chapter) was 3/4. She indicated that though she had tried to cut down on her drinking, she used alcohol daily for pain control and to help her sleep. She did not begin to use alcohol heavily until her retirement when her disability began and her marital tensions increased. At the time of our evaluation, she was drinking over a half pint of whiskey per day.

What are the cognitive strengths and weaknesses?

There is no evidence of a frank dementia on the neuropsychological evaluation. This case is challenging in that despite her stated years of education, Ms. H's reading score, used to estimate her premorbid level of functioning, was in the low average range. The NSRP norms were thus utilized for Ms. H. Memory functioning appeared within normal limits on the Fuld, and although initial recall was poor on the Logical Memory I, retention was at 75 percent 30 minutes later. Deficits were apparent in visuospatial tasks and on tasks of mental flexibility. Compared to normative data, Ms. H scored in the unimpaired range on the VFD but in the impaired range on the Hooper and Controlled Oral Word tests.

What practical recommendations can be made?

Ms. H was educated to the effects of alcohol abuse during older age and was told that she could not drive until she passed a driver's evaluation with a road test. There were no other recommendations made regarding her ability to live independently or perform IADLs.

CASE #10: MR. H

Mr. H was a 79-year-old, widowed, African-American male who presented to the hospital after falling on the ice and breaking his hip. During the hospital stay, he developed delirium tremens, a dangerous syndrome associated with alcohol withdrawal. This was managed by Ativan. Other medical problems included gastritis and chronic obstructive pulmonary disease. Mr. H had a history of heavy drinking for 45 years. He had worked in an auto factory and completed eight years of education. He was reportedly completing all of his own ADL and IADL care. He was referred for a neuropsychological evaluation to see if he was cognitively capable of returning to independent living. Testing was completed one month subsequent to the delirium tremens. The results of the evaluation were as follows:
WRAT-R Reading (scaled score) 44
Dementia Rating Scale (total) 122
Attention 34
Initiation/Perseveration 29
Construction 6
Conceptualization 37
Memory 16
Logical Memory I 11
Logical Memory II 3
Boston Naming Test 26

Fuld Storage 31
Fuld Retrieval 18
Fuld Repeated Retrieval 6
Fuld Ineffective Reminders 15
Visual Form Discrimination 12
Hooper VOT 9.5
Controlled Oral Word Test 18

Is there evidence of cerebral dysfunction?

Mr. H's profile is consistent with a presentation of dementia. Memory scores are significantly impaired on both the Logical Memory and Fuld tests.

What are cognitive strengths and weaknesses?

In the case of Logical Memory, although Mr. H's immediate recall is better than Ms. H's (as per case #9), his retention is only 27 percent after a 30-minute delay. Scores on visuospatial and mental flexibility tests are also in the severely impaired range.

What practical recommendations can be made?

Based upon the severity of his cognitive deficits, it was recommended that Mr. H not be allowed to return to living alone.

SUMMARY

In health care settings, unlike Alzheimer's centers or National Institutes of Mental Health (NIMH) research units, cases are not selected out. All types of etiologies of dementia and delirium are encountered. The purpose of this chapter was to demonstrate some of the broad-based applications that the NSRP test battery can have with older adults. The cases are presented as illustrations, not as generalizations.

Chapter 7

Behavioral Treatment
of Geriatric Depression
in Health Care Settings

Our adaptation of the Lewinsohnian model of depression is unique in that non-mental health professionals serve as the primary treater of depression. In our validity study, trained occupational therapists were used to treat depression in a geriatric rehabilitation setting. This method of treatment was found highly effective in reducing symptoms of depression and was associated with high patient satisfaction with the treatment program.

This treatment is designed to occur concomitantly with other standard treatments, such as an occupational, physical, or speech therapy session in a rehabilitation program or in long-term care settings. For example, it might be morning activities of daily living care. The treatment consists of the following elements:

1. Provision of a rationale for the treatment in which patients are taught that what they do is related to how they feel
2. Explanation of the goal of increasing positive events and decreasing negative ones
3. Relaxation and mood monitoring
4. Daily incorporation of pleasant events into the hospital schedule
5. Reinforcement for functional gains

Depression treatment includes four components:

1. Relaxation
2. Mood monitoring

3. Pleasant Event scheduling
4. Reinforcement for functional gains

SPECIFIC METHODS OF DETECTION AND TREATMENT

Upon admission to a hospital, rehabilitation, or long-term care unit, a patient is greeted, welcomed to the facility, and administered the Geriatric Depression Scale (Brink et al., 1982) within 24 hours. We recommend that the clinician read the items on the scale to the patient and record his or her responses directly on the score sheet. The scale is scored according to cutoffs that have been validated by empirical research. A score of greater than 10 is considered to be significant. If patients score above the cutoff for depression they are told about the treatment for depression and asked if they would care to receive such services. Once they agree, depression treatment starts the very next day.

ORGANIZATION OF EACH SESSION

In order to maintain an acceptable degree of consistency in each session, it is necessary to establish a standard approach to follow with each patient. This will ensure that any differences in patient outcome can be attributed to factors that are most likely beyond the control of the clinician and will facilitate valid quantitative analysis of outcome. For example, a patient's mood might be influenced by their success or failure during regular occupational therapy (OT). If we measured mood some days after therapy and other days after administration of the pleasant events schedule, it would add a level of uncertainty to outcome.

We recommend that individual therapy be scheduled for 90 minutes. During the first 20 minutes and last 20 minutes of each session, the therapist should conduct a variety of behavioral treatment interventions. The session should be organized as follows:

• Mood rating
• Relaxation treatment
• Pleasant event

- Mood rating
- Goal setting
- OT Treatment
- Graphing progress
- Mood Rating

#1: *Mood Monitoring*

According to Lewinsohn, Hoberman, and Clark (1989), "The central theoretical construct of behavioral theories of depression has been that relatively low rates of positive experiences ... constitute a critical antecedent for the occurrence of depression. Thus, mood was viewed as a function of the relative balance of positive and negative experiences" (p. 472). It is a well-established finding that there is a high correlation between the number of pleasant activities an individual engages in and an individual's mood. (Lewinsohn and Talkington, 1979; Teri and Uomoto, 1991). Consequently, an important component of this treatment program is the daily evaluation of each patient's mood in order to determine the association between the various behavioral interventions used by the clinical staff and patients' perception of how they feel. Thus, we recommend the therapist monitor mood at three predetermined periods during the depression intervention portion of each treatment session. The good news is that mood monitoring is a relatively simple procedure that will take a minimum amount of time. A ten-point analog scale is used to record how a patient feels at a given point during each treatment session.

Procedure

Patients will be provided with an analog mood rating scale three times during each session. Instructions to the patient are as follows:

I would like you to take a moment to indicate on this scale how you are feeling right now. As you can see, it is a 10-point scale. Please circle the number that best describes how you feel right now.

1	2	3	4	5	6	7	8	9	10
Worst I've									Best I've
ever felt									ever felt

#2: Relaxation: Controlled Breathing

Slowing down and controlling breathing has been shown to reduce anxiety and, thus, reduce the unpleasantness of a situation. Various breathing techniques have been used alone or in combination with progressive muscle relaxation to reduce stress. Deep, diaphragmatic breathing is inconsistent with anxiety and stress. It can be taught by having patients lie down or sit back in a chair, placing their hands on their abdomen, and exhaling so that their lungs are empty of air. Then, they are asked to inhale deeply and to try to direct the air to the area where their hands are (Phillips, 1988). Generally, tension and anxiety can be reduced simply by having patients inhale and exhale evenly to a count of four (i.e., take in air for four seconds, let it out for four seconds, etc.).

Imagery

Creating and thinking about an image of a peaceful, pleasant scene is inconsistent with distress and can also distract the patient from thinking about stressors. This activity is believed to bring about a calm, relaxed mental state. Used alone or in conjunction with progressive muscle relaxation, imagery can greatly enhance the relaxation obtained. Therapists can assist the imagery process by suggesting that the patient think about calm, enjoyable times from the past, or, if the patient has difficulty, suggesting a typical experience such as lying on a beach with the noise of waves in the background, etc. The patient should be encouraged to completely involve him or herself in the image, concentrating on the details and trying to fill his or her mind with the experience of the image (Blanchard and Andrasik, 1985).

Patients may need a great deal of encouragement and reinforcement for their efforts throughout the sessions. Include these exercises in the goal-setting component of treatment and plan for successes, which you then may reinforce liberally. For example, scenes of favorite vacation or recreation spots can help induce a relaxed state. Monitor how well patients can visualize these scenes and how relaxed they feel.

Directions for Controlled Breathing with Imagery

The session should begin with the induction of relaxation with controlled breathing techniques. When breathing is well established, the patient can continue breathing properly while focusing on imagery. The last five minutes will be spent on relaxing imagery.

All instructions to the patient should be spoken in a slow, quiet voice, with a short pause between sentences. Therapists should model a relaxed state for the patient.

First session only. Explain to the patient the purpose and rationale of the treatments with the following statement:

> The aim of this breathing control method is to slow down your breathing into deep, steady, paced breaths, which will help you relax by automatically calming you down. When a person is excited, upset, or under stress, their breathing is automatically fast, shallow, and sometimes uneven. When you take control of your breathing and return it to being deep, steady, and paced, you can help yourself become more calm and relaxed.

Step 1:

> Direct the patient to assume a comfortable position, such as lying on a mat or bed. Let the patient direct you as to what he or she finds most comfortable. Have him or her close his or her eyes and keep them closed as much as possible. Take a few moments for both of you to get as comfortable as you can.

Step 2:

> Begin controlled breathing. Have the patient place his or her hands on the abdomen, and exhale so that his or her lungs are empty of air. Then ask the patient to inhale deeply and to try to direct the air to the area where his or her hands are (Phillips, 1988). Maintain focus on the breathing as long as needed for the patient to acquire a smooth, even, consistent rate of breathing.

Encourage the patient to relax his or her chest and allow air to fill the lungs, as evidenced by his or her stomach rising. If there are problems, demonstrate the breathing yourself.

Keep the patient breathing consistently in this manner for three minutes before continuing on with the imagery, so that the patient can focus on the exercises and still maintain good breathing. (This will become easier with practice).

Step 3:

Say, "Now I would like you to imagine a relaxing, calm, happy scene in your mind. It can be something from your own experience, or an image that seems quiet and relaxing to you, such as lying on your favorite beach. Do you have a scene in mind?"

If the patient says "yes," continue.

If the patient says "no," then suggest a few images for the patient, allowing a few seconds in between suggestions for the patient to try to imagine them. In some cases, you may need to keep giving them images to focus on throughout the procedure. Images such as lying on a beach or a hillside are good.

Try to imagine the sights, sounds, and smells of the place. Think about how it feels to be in the place. Imagine that you are totally relaxed, that your muscles are hanging loosely on you and unmoving.

Pause for a few moments, allowing the patient to concentrate. Watch for evidence of problems keeping the image in mind, etc. Feel free to frequently ask the patient if they have the image in mind, or ask if they want you to suggest one.

Keeping the image in mind, think about how nice it is to be here, and focus on the relaxed feeling of being here.

pause

Are your thoughts calm?

If the patient says yes, continue.

If the patient says no, ask him or her what place he or she is imagining, and what kinds of thoughts he or she is having. If these are problematic for trying to relax, then shift to making suggestions about what to imagine.

Keep focusing on your peaceful place, and on how you feel while you are there.

For the rest of the five-minute period, keep making statements as above to help the patient maintain peaceful imagery and a relaxed state. Be observant for discomfort or inattention, which may interfere with the imagery.

Listed below are ideas for imagery that were well received by older adults:

1. Boat ride
2. Walking through the park, nature trail, neighborhood, or own backyard
3. Shopping at the mall
4. Riding on a motorcycle
5. Visiting grandchildren
6. A ride in a glider
7. People-watching at the mall
8. A trip to Hawaii, hometown, friend's home
9. Sitting in favorite chair reminiscing
10. Planning a special event (retirement party, birthday, etc.)

#3. Pleasant Events Schedule

The Pleasant Events Schedule will help to identify daily events that are pleasurable to the patient. Depressed patients often stop engaging in these pleasant activities. In session #1, you will administer the Pleasant Events Schedule. From that schedule you can then identify events that you can engage in during future sessions (e.g., reading newspapers, puzzles, cards, etc.). The events used in treatment will be individualized based on responses to the Pleasant Events Schedule. The Pleasant Events Schedule is an adaptation of the one authored by Teri and Logsdon (1991). Ten items from that scale were dropped since they referred to around-the-house activities or outings to special locations.

Directions (to be read to the patient): This schedule contains a list of events or activities that people sometimes enjoy. It is designed to find out about things you have enjoyed doing in the past. Because this list contains events or activities that might happen to a wide variety of people, you may find that many of the items have not happened to you in the past. It is not expected that anyone will have done all of these things. There are no right or wrong answers. Circle YES if the event is one you have enjoyed in the past. Circle NO if you have not enjoyed the event.

PLEASANT EVENTS SCHEDULE

Pleasant Events	Have you enjoyed this event in the past?	
1. Being outside	YES	NO
2. Meeting someone new or making new friends	YES	NO
3. Planning trips or vacations, looking at travel brochures, or traveling	YES	NO
4. Reading or listening to stories, novels, plays, or poems	YES	NO
5. Listening to music (radio, stereo)	YES	NO
6. Watching TV	YES	NO
7. Thinking about something good in the future	YES	NO
8. Completing a difficult task	YES	NO
9. Laughing	YES	NO
10. Doing jigsaw puzzles, crosswords, and word games	YES	NO
11. Having meals with friends or family	YES	NO

12. Taking a shower or bath . . . .   YES   NO

13. Listening to nonmusic radio programs (talk
    shows) . . . .   YES   NO

14. Making or eating snacks . . . .   YES   NO

15. Combing or brushing your hair . . . .   YES   NO

16. Taking a nap . . . .   YES   NO

17. Being with my family . . . .   YES   NO

18. Wearing certain clothes (such as new, informal,
    formal, or favorite clothes) . . . .   YES   NO

19. Listening to the sound of nature (birdsong,
    wind, surf) . . . .   YES   NO

20. Having friends come to visit . . . .   YES   NO

21. Getting/sending letters, cards, or notes . . . . . .   YES   NO

22. Watching the clouds, the sky, or a storm . . . . .   YES   NO

23. Going on outings (to the park, a picnic, a bar-
    becue, etc.) . . . .   YES   NO

24. Reading, watching, or listening to the news . .   YES   NO

25. Watching people . . . .   YES   NO

26. Having coffee, tea, a soda, etc., with friends . .   YES   NO

27. Being complimented or told I have done some-
    thing well . . . .   YES   NO

28. Being told I am loved . . . .   YES   NO

29. Having family members or friends tell me
    something that makes me proud of them . . . . .   YES   NO

30. Seeing or speaking with old friends (in person,
    or on the telephone) . . . .   YES   NO

31. Looking at the stars or the moon . . . .   YES   NO

32. Playing cards or games . . . .   YES   NO

33. Doing handiwork (crocheting, woodworking, crafts, knitting, painting, drawing, ceramics, clay work, or other) .... YES   NO

34. Exercising (walking, aerobics, swimming, dancing, or other) .... YES   NO

35. Indoor gardening or related activities (tending plants) .... YES   NO

36. Going to museums, art exhibits, or related cultural activities .... YES   NO

37. Looking at photo albums and photos .... YES   NO

38. Stamp collecting or other collections .... YES   NO

39. Going for a ride in the car .... YES   NO

40. Going to church, attending religious ceremonies .... YES   NO

41. Singing .... YES   NO

42. Grooming yourself (wearing makeup, having your hair done) .... YES   NO

43. Recalling and discussing past events .... YES   NO

44. Participating in or watching sports .... YES   NO

Have we missed any?   Please write them in below.

Has there been any change in your life that affected how you responded to the scale?   What was it?

THE RESPONSES FROM THE PLEASANT EVENTS SCHEDULE ARE USED TO DETERMINE WHICH ACTIVITIES WILL BE ENGAGED IN DURING TREATMENT SESSIONS.

#4 Providing Reinforcement

Depressed patients often perceive themselves as doing nothing right. They do not notice the gains they are making. In order to underscore their progress, reinforcement and graphing of progress will be a daily part of treatment.

Reinforcement Menu

- Social Reinforcement (Praise)—most powerful
- Percent effort in therapy (graph)
- Time spent on task (graph)
- Functional Improvement gains (graph)
- Improvement in mood ratings (graph)

We recommend that therapists record each day's activities on a daily record sheet, as this will help ensure that the treatment described above is being followed in the proper order and being completed correctly.

DEPRESSION TREATMENT PROJECT

Daily Treatment Record

Date:_____ Patient Name:_____

Clinician:_____

1. MOOD RATING

1   2   3   4   5   6   7   8   9   10
Worst I've   Best I've
ever felt   ever felt

2. RELAXATION COMPLETED   [Yes]   [No]

3. PLEASANT EVENTS

1.

.

2.

___

3.

___

4. MOOD RATING

___

  1   2   3   4   5   6   7   8   9   10
Worst I've   Best I've
ever felt   ever felt

5. TREATMENT

___

___

___

6. REINFORCEMENT USED

  1.

  ___

  2.

  ___

  3.

  ___

7. MOOD RATING

___

  1   2   3   4   5   6   7   8   9   10
Worst I've   Best I've
ever felt   ever felt

CASE EXAMPLES

Ms. G

Ms. G was a 65-year-old, retired, divorced, African American who underwent a right knee replacement due to severe joint disease from arthritis. She lived alone, had completed six years of education in rural Alabama, and functioned independently in her activities of daily living before her surgery. Cognitive testing revealed that her functioning was within normal limits on tests of attention, language, memory, visuospatial skills, and mental flexibility when compared to individuals of the same age and education level. However, she reported moderate levels of depression on the Geriatric Depression Scale (GDS = 15), with complaints of feeling helpless, hopeless, and worthless. She was immediately entered into the behavioral treatment protocol. Ms. G had an eleven-day length of stay and completed nine behavioral treatment sessions. Upon admission, she required assistance with the following activities of daily living: bathing, upper extremity dressing, lower extremity dressing, and tub transfers.

Her pleasant events inventory revealed that she enjoyed many activities. These were incorporated into her daily treatment, including reminiscing about family, reading scriptures, listening to classical music, enjoying a glass of cola, reading the paper, relaxing in a lounge chair, and planning a shopping trip. By the end of her rehabilitation treatment, her depression score was reduced to the nondepressed range (GDS = 7) and she was independent in all but one of her activities of daily living. Graphs were used to demonstrate to Ms. G her functional progress.

Ms. S

Ms. S entered the rehabilitation hospital after suffering from a pulmonary embolism, and due to peripheral vascular disease became too weakened to be discharged immediately home where she lived alone. She was a 71-year-old, widowed, retired press operator who upon admission to the rehabilitation program scored a 15/30 on the Geriatric Depression Scale (moderately depressed range). Upon admission, she required physical assistance with all ADLs including feeding, grooming, dressing, and transferring.

The Pleasant Events inventory indicated that Ms. S enjoyed a number of things including meeting new people, reminiscing, combing her hair, reading, handiwork, as well as a number of other activities. In all, Ms. S completed eight sessions. Pleasant events incorporated into the therapies included listening to music, tending to plants, sewing, reading and discussing short stories, talking about friends, planning a trip, and reading the newspaper and discussing news items. Mood ratings indicated a linear trend from sad to happy over the course of the treatments. Graphs demonstrated to Ms. S her improvement with mood corresponding with her involvement with pleasurable activities.

Prior to discharge, Ms. S's mood and physical abilities were measured again. Ms. S scored a 10/30 on the Geriatric Depression Scale, a decrease from her admission score, moving her to the borderline range of depression. Upon completion of her rehabilitation stay, Ms. S no longer required any physical assistance with her ADL skills and was fully independent in feeding, grooming, bathing, and dressing. Ms. S also reported being very satisfied with the behavioral treatment program.

Chapter 8

Detection and Treatment of Alcohol Abuse

Alcoholism is a serious health problem in the nation's elderly. Alcoholism is the third leading killer of adults in the United States (Benshoff and Roberto, 1987) and is the third most common psychiatric diagnosis in elderly men (Ticehurst, 1990). Schuckit and Pastor (1978) found that elderly alcohol abusers typically present to medical/surgical units with problems. In a survey of 113 consecutive VA admissions, 20 percent of men met the criteria for alcoholism, with 9 percent actively drinking. Brody (1982) estimated that 10 to 15 percent of elderly seeking attention in a medical office abuse alcohol. Curtis et al. (1989) surveyed 417 consecutive admissions to the Johns Hopkins Hospital, using standardized screening instruments. Overall, 21 percent of those over age 60 were abusing alcohol.

Studies on the prevalence of alcoholism in the elderly have revealed two types of alcoholics: early and late onset (Brody, 1982; Zimberg, 1984). Two-thirds of elderly alcoholics are represented in the early onset group. These individuals have had longstanding alcoholic histories that continued into later life. The more severe long-term effects of alcohol (discussed in a later section) are more likely in this group. The late onset alcoholics developed their drinking problem in later life. Authors have hypothesized various stressors associated with late onset alcoholism, and these include depression, bereavement, retirement, loneliness, physical illness, and pain. Both groups are thought, however, to respond to the same type of treatment.

Stroke, both hemorrhagic and occlusive, is the most common diagnostic group of the elderly in the inpatient rehabilitation setting, with hypertension being the strongest predictor of all forms of stroke. In a prospective study of cardiovascular disease, the risk of hemorrhagic stroke more than doubled for "light" drinkers and nearly tripled for "heavy" drinkers, independent of hypertensive status and other risk factors (Donahue et al., 1986). No significant relationships were noted between alcohol use and thromboembolic stroke. The pathogenesis of this relationship is unknown but may include the association between alcohol and atrial fibrillation (Wolf et al., 1978), alteration in platelet metabolism and function (Haut and Cowan, 1974) and/or weakening of the cerebral arteries (Donahue et al., 1986). When individuals' alcohol consumption was reduced, the risk of developing hemorrhagic stroke was lowered as compared to those whose intake remained the same or increased. Thus, accurate identification and treatment of alcohol abuse in the elderly within rehabilitation is critical to maximize prevention of disability, to understand the influence of alcohol in the etiology of disability, and to enhance functional outcomes.

DEFINING ALCOHOLISM

Alcoholism in the elderly is often hidden due to its subtle presentation. Nevertheless, Beresford et al. (1988) described four aspects of the addiction to alcohol.

The first aspect, *Tolerance,* refers to the alcoholic's need to increase drinking by 50 percent in order to achieve the same effect. For example, a man who had four drinks a day may find himself, over time, drinking a pint or two. Typically, the alcoholic is seeking a feeling of escape and drinks until this feeling is acquired.

The second aspect, *Withdrawal,* refers to physical symptoms that follow six to twelve hours after the blood alcohol level has decreased. Common symptoms include increased blood pressure, low grade fever, sweating, tremors, nausea, and increased anxiety. Beresford and colleagues (1988) are quick to point out that other medications, particularly antianxiety medicines and other sedatives, mask the withdrawal syndrome. They also caution that total withdrawal from alcohol can be very dangerous and needs to be monitored closely by medical personnel.

The third aspect, *Loss of control* over the drinking behavior and preoccupation with guilt and shame, is the most subtle aspect of the diagnosis. Often, this loss of control leads to severe loneliness and isolation. This phenomenon can be observed in alcoholics that begin an evening determined to have one drink and end up becoming drunk.

Finally, *Social decline* and the loss, or at least the severe straining, of familial and other close relationships is the last aspect of this definition. Therefore, it is important to carefully assess the patient's psychosocial history, both prior to and after the onset of the alcoholism.

Maletta (1982) grouped drinking problems into several categories when defining alcoholism. These overlap significantly with the definition by Beresford and his colleagues. The five categories were (1) symptoms that developed as a result of drinking (e.g., blackouts, tremors); (2) psychological dependence and health problems related to alcohol use; (3) problems with relatives, colleagues, friends, or neighbors related to alcohol use; (4) problems with employment or finances; and (5) problems with law enforcement officials. The label "problem drinking" is applicable to people who exhibit behaviors from more than one of the listed categories.

The Diagnostic and Statistical Manual of Mental Disorders (DSM-IV) criteria for psychoactive substance dependence requires at least three of seven criteria (DSM-IV, 1994). However, these criteria do not consider the effect of alcohol on aging physiology, nor do they include the commonly presenting physical complications of chronic alcohol ingestion in the elderly. Many elderly drinkers develop physical problems with alcohol because of age-related physiological changes, concurrent medications, or disease-impaired organ function (Scott and Mitchell, 1988). In addition, the criteria do not take into account the psychosocial and occupational differences in seniors compared to younger people. As confusion persists in diagnosis for the elderly, Rains and Ditzler (1993) delineated the following cautions in the use of the DSM-IV criteria in the elderly:

1. Development of Marked Tolerance

Because of increased cellular sensitivity, reverse tolerance may occur with alcohol consumption either remaining the same or reduced in the elderly. Multiple medical problems coupled with polypharmacy often result in intolerable drug interactions or side effects, precluding increased intake. Consequently, the development of tolerance is increasingly difficult to recognize.

2. Characteristic Withdrawal Symptoms When Substance Is Withheld

Due to decreased volume of distribution and increased sensitivity to alcohol, hazardous consumption is lower for the elderly. No data is available as to whether withdrawal symptoms occur, or are recognizable, when alcohol intake is low. Heavy drinkers will certainly have withdrawal symptoms, but the difficulty comes in recognizing the cause. Delirium is a common presentation in the frail elderly. Clinically, the hyperautonomic arousal associated with delirium is often indistinguishable from DTs or alcoholic hallucinosis, making etiologic inferences difficult. Also, polypharmacy may result in cross-tolerance, which permits the cessation of drinking without the clinical presentation of withdrawal.

3. Substance Taken Longer or in Larger Amounts Than Intended

As increased cellular sensitivity results in a decreased threshold for organ toxicity, alcohol consumption may be self-limited by physical symptoms of alcohol toxicity. Thus, loss of control when drinking is not typically seen in the elderly.

4. Persistent Desire or Unsuccessful Attempts to Control Use

Elderly drinkers may not attempt to quit or cut down their consumption as they, as well as their physicians and family, may misattribute the signs, symptoms, and sequelae of alcoholism to the aging process or related to other medical problems. Even when symptoms are identified, denial of the problem occurs, with drinkers citing survival into late life as evidence of their invulnerability to the disease.

5. Large Amounts of Time Expended Getting, Taking, and Recovering from the Substance

With an increased peak blood concentration in the elderly for any given amount of alcohol consumed, greater effects are achieved from smaller quantities. Thus, elderly alcoholics may drink less over time rather than more, and spend less time obtaining and consuming alcohol.

6. Social, Occupational, or Recreational Activities Given Up

As the elderly, in general, often give up previously enjoyed activities due to chronic medical problems that interfere with daily life and function, it is more difficult to discern the specific role of alcohol in limiting these activities. Family and work obligations are also significantly decreased for the elderly with changed family roles, responsibilities, and retirement. Thus, periods of intoxication or withdrawal may not demonstrably interfere with work or family obligations.

7. Continued Use Despite Knowledge of Problems Caused by Substances

A decline in psychosocial and physiologic function is often normal for the elderly population. Because alcohol-related problems may be misattributed to causes other than drinking, the older person's drinking is less likely to be challenged and consumption continues.

In an effort to effectively incorporate the elderly and the concept of a threshold for hazardous consumption into the DSM-IV diagnostic schema for alcohol dependence, Rains, Ditzler, and Blanchette (1989) suggest an epidemiologically guided definition of alcoholism in the elderly oriented toward a threshold for morbid risk rather than a reference criterion of consumption, as often used in diagnosing alcoholism. Willenbring (1988) suggests that because of increased sensitivity to alcohol, medical problems for the elderly may be caused or exacerbated by regular consumption as low as one standard drink per day or two to three standard drinks per occasion frequently repeated. Curtis et al. (1989) found only 11 percent of alcohol-positive elderly consumed five drinks per day as compared to 40 percent of younger patients. Further research is needed to determine the consumption threshold detrimental to the average elderly person.

DETECTION OF ALCOHOL ABUSE
IN HEALTH CARE SETTINGS

Curtis et al. (1989) also investigated physician detection of the alcohol abuse. Forty-five percent of nonelderly were correctly identified by physicians, whereas only 27 percent of elderly alcohol abusers were correctly identified. Gender effects were evident in that no elderly women were diagnosed alcoholic by the house officer! The authors concluded that routine screening instruments are needed. Similarly, Schuckit et al. (1980) found that physicians failed to detect 90 percent of elderly alcoholics in their sample.

Lichtenberg et al. (1993) examined the relationship of alcohol abuse in older urban medical patients to both age and sex. Detection of alcohol abuse by physicians and nurses was also examined. The sample consisted of 150 consecutive admissions, 60 percent women and 66 percent African American. Two-thirds of the sample were above the age of 75 years. Alcohol abuse was assessed by the CAGE questionnaire (to be reviewed shortly), and a rater, blind to the study, reviewed the chart for notations about alcohol use or abuse. Overall, 17 percent of the sample scored greater than 2 on the CAGE. Men had a significantly higher rate of alcohol abuse than did women (Chi Square = 9.42, p <.05). Those individuals aged 60 to 74 years had a significantly higher rate of alcohol abuse than did those over age 75 (see Table 8.1 for details). Detection of alcohol abuse varied by the patient's sex. Whereas 50 percent of the men scoring above the CAGE cutoff were detected by physicians or nurses, none of the women reporting alcohol abuse symptoms on the CAGE were detected.

TABLE 8.1. Prevalence of Alcohol Abuse in Medically Ill Elderly Men and Women

	Women	Men
Young-old (Ages 60 to 74)	17% (n = 30)	48% (n = 27)
Old-old (Ages 75+)	3% (n = 60)	15% (n = 33)

ASSESSMENT OF ALCOHOLISM

Hanks and Lichtenberg (1996) furthered research on the relationship between alcohol abuse and age by increasing the sample to 812 participants, ages 60 to 103 years old. Once again, age was significantly related to CAGE scores, with older individuals reporting fewer symptoms of alcohol abuse than younger individuals. Whereas rates for alcohol abuse were 21 percent for those ages 60 to 69, and 17 percent for those ages 70 to 79, rates were only 6 percent and 11 percent for those 80 to 89 and 90 to 103 years, respectively.

Detecting alcoholism depends upon the health care staff learning the subtle cluster of symptoms that are present in older alcoholics. In their early study, Rosin and Glatt (1971) investigated the consequences of alcohol excess in the elderly. Only 1 of the 36 patients suffered from delirium tremens, a common withdrawal symptom in younger adults; 66 percent, however, displayed self-neglect, 33 percent displayed falls, 31 percent had confusion, 11 percent aggressiveness, and 56 percent had their family relationships terminated. Not all of the above problems, however, were due to alcohol abuse. Indeed, many of these problems are experienced by a considerable number of non-alcohol-abusing elderly. Nevertheless, observing a constellation of these problems may help to detect alcohol abuse. In Table 8.2 the common nonspecific presentations of alcohol abuse in the elderly are noted (Atkinson and Kofoed, 1982; Hartford and Damorajski, 1982; Ticehurst, 1990; Wattis, 1981).

TABLE 8.2. Nonspecific Presentations of Alcohol Abuse in the Elderly

---

General Health:
Poor grooming, incontinence, myopathy, falling, accidental hypothermia, seizures, malnutrition, diarrhea, unexplained bruises or burns, peptic-ulceration, heart and liver disease, chronic obstructive pulmonary disease

Interpersonal:
Confusion, aggression, termination of family relationships

Alcohol:
Preoccupation with drinking, rapid intake, alcohol used as medicine, using alcohol alone, protecting alcohol supply

---

As can be seen in the table, behaviors are separated into three categories: general health, interpersonal changes, and alcohol-related behaviors. The list of health problems common in the elderly alcoholic is a lengthy one. The more obvious problems and ones that should raise the clinician's suspicions include poor grooming; presentation with unexplained falls, bruises, or burns; and malnutrition. Other common problems in this group that can be obtained through laboratory examination are heart problems, liver disease, seizures, chronic obstructive pulmonary disease, accidental hypothermia, and peptic ulcer disease (Atkinson and Kofoed, 1982; Ticehurst, 1990). Alcohol abuse is one of several conditions to rule out when a patient presents with symptoms of dementia. Wattis (1981) reported on seven cases of alcoholism that were initially undetected. In one case, an 81-year-old woman was admitted to the hospital with her daughter stating that her mother suffered memory problems and frequent falling only, of course, for the clinician to find out that she drank heavy quantities of wine and scotch each day. Hartford and Damorajski (1982) found that 28 percent of dementia patients had undiagnosed alcoholism.

Interpersonal changes are another area for clinicians to assess in the elderly. As mentioned in the previous section on definition of the disease, social decline is part of alcoholism. This is often displayed by aggression and hostility toward family members, especially when the topic of alcohol is addressed. Rosin and Glatt (1971), in their early study, found that 56 percent of elderly alcoholics had at least one family relationship terminated by their drinking.

Intermittent and unexplained periods of confusion are also classic signs of alcohol abuse.

The alcoholic's relationship with the alcohol is another area of diagnostic importance (see Table 8.2). Alcohol sometimes replaces other people in the role of comforter and supporter, and, thus, alcoholics protect their alcohol supply. The alcoholic often hides the alcohol as a function of denial. Alcohol is sometimes used as medicine to decrease pain and discomfort. Alcoholics are preoccupied with their drinking. This preoccupation causes them to use alcohol alone, and to rapidly ingest the alcohol.

USE OF SCREENING MEASURES
TO DETECT ALCOHOLISM

Curtis et al. (1989), in their diagnostic study, concluded that the routine use of screening instruments is needed in order to more accurately detect alcoholism in the elderly. Two screening measures will be discussed here (see Tables 8.3 and 8.4).

The CAGE Questionnaire (see Table 8.3), described by its author (Ewing, 1984), was developed in 1970 and is a most efficient and effective screening device. The questionnaire is made up of four simple questions about attitudes and behaviors related to an individual's drinking. A score of two affirmative responses raises the suspicion of alcoholism, whereas a score of three of four affirmative responses is almost always a sure sign of alcoholism. The original data gathered on the CAGE consisted of comparing responses of sixteen alcoholics with 114 nonalcoholic randomly selected medical patients. A second study of 166 male alcoholics revealed the CAGE to be a valid screening instrument with a sensitivity of 85 percent and specificity of 100 percent. Bush et al. (1987) prospectively studied 518 patients admitted to the orthopedic and medical services of a community-based hospital during a six-month period. The criterion measure used for alcohol abuse was the standard criteria from the Diagnostic and Statistical Manual, Third Edition (DSM-III). The CAGE and three laboratory tests were compared for their ability to detect alcohol abuse. The laboratory tests were very insensitive, whereas the CAGE questionnaire was highly valid. The CAGE had a sensitivity of 85 percent and specificity of 89

TABLE 8.3. Alcohol Screening Measure: CAGE Questionnaire

C—Have you ever felt you ought to Cut down on your drinking? (Y)

A—Have people Annoyed you by criticizing your drinking? (Y)

G—Have you ever felt bad or Guilty about your drinking? (Y)

E—Have you ever had a drink first thing in the morning to steady your nerves or get rid of a hangover (Eye-opener)? (Y)

CAGE SCORE < or = 2: suspicion of alcoholism

TABLE 8.4. Alcohol Screening Measure: BMAST Questionnaire

Brief Michigan Alcohol Screening Test

---

1. Do you feel you are a normal drinker? (N)
2. Do friends and relatives think you are normal drinker? (N)
3. Have you ever attended Alcoholics Anonymous (AA)? (Y)
4. Have you ever lost friends or girlfriends/boyfriends because of drinking? (Y)
5. Have you ever gotten into trouble at work because of drinking? (Y)
6. Have you ever neglected your obligations, your family, or your work for two or more days in a row because you were drinking? (Y)
7. Have you ever had delirium tremens (DTs), severe shaking, heard voices, or seen things that weren't there after heavy drinking? (Y)
8. Have you ever gone to anyone for help about your drinking? (Y)
9. Have you ever been in a hospital because of drinking? (Y)
10. Have you ever been arrested for drunk driving after drinking? (Y)

BMAST > 4: suspicion of alcoholism

---

percent. Curtis et al. (1989) found the CAGE to be highly useful in detecting elderly alcohol abusers.

The Michigan Alcohol Screening Test (MAST), a 25-item instrument, was developed to provide a consistent and quantifiable method to detect alcoholism (Hedlund and Vieweg, 1984; Selzer, 1971). All questions are presented in a yes/no format. Pokorney, Miller, and Kaplan (1972) selected 10 out of the 25 questions and developed the Brief Michigan Alcohol Screening Test (BMAST) (see Table 8.4). Internal consistency for the BMAST was reported at .80 and .60 on samples of all age alcoholics. Willenbring et al. (1987) conducted an investigation of the MAST and its various short forms in a study aimed at screening for alcoholism in the elderly. They compared 52 consecutive older adults (age>60) admitted to a Veterans' Administration alcohol treatment program with 33 controls (nonalcoholics) admitted for medical reasons. The BMAST was the best of all short MAST forms in detecting alcoholism in the sample. When using a cutoff score of four, the BMAST had a sensitivity rate of 91 percent and a specificity rate of 83 percent. Age and education were not significantly correlated with BMAST scores.

Despite accurate and brief assessment instruments, there appear to be many reasons why health care professionals fail to recognize alcohol abuse in older adults. These include the widespread belief in many myths that persist about alcohol abuse in older adults.

Myth #1: Drinking (in the elderly) won't hurt them.

As can be seem in Table 8.5, alcohol has many toxic effects on its elderly abusers. Since alcohol affects so many parts of the body, discussing them is often viewed as an "organ recital"! Thienhaus and Hartford (1984) described the physical changes that affect the distribution of alcohol in an older adult. At age 25, for example, 61 percent of the human body is composed of water, but by age 70, this percentage drops to 53 percent. Because alcohol is rapidly distributed through the body water compartment after ingestion, less alcohol is needed by an older adult to produce acute intoxication. In addition, decreases in liver and kidney function result in alcohol remaining in the body longer (Gomberg, 1990; Benshoff and Roberto, 1987). Alcohol, when abused, is a killer. In the elderly, alcohol kills from chronic debilitating and deteriorating conditions rather than from acute events. Thienhaus and Hartford (1984) concluded that the aging body is more susceptible to the toxic effects of alcohol. As can be seen in Table 8.5, alcoholism produces damage to the central nervous system, the gastrointestinal system, and the cardio-vascular system. The most common problems are cirrhosis of the liver, pancreatitis, heart dysfunction, and neurologic damage.

Eckardt and Martin (1986) estimated that 50 to 70 percent of elderly alcoholics have cognitive impairment and that 9 percent develop severe dementia. They cited visuospatial functioning and abstract reasoning as the most consistently impaired areas of cognitive functioning. Hubbard, Santos, and Santos (1979) stated that almost a quarter of elderly alcohol abusers presented to the hospital as functionally senile. When the patients were withdrawn from

TABLE 8.5. Physical Problems Associated with Alcoholism in the Elderly

---

Benshoff and Roberto (1987):

1. *Neurologic:* Peripheral neuropathy, cerebellar degeneration, sleep disturbances, sexual dysfunction

2. *Gastrointestinal:* Cirrhosis of the liver, pancreatitis (pain, nausea, vomiting), upper respiratory infections, stomach, colon problems

3. *Cardiovascular:* Exacerbation of all heart problems

Eckhardt and Martin (1986):

1. *Brain Dysfunction:* 50 to 70 percent alcoholics have cognitive impairment; 90 percent develop severe dementia.

Hubbard, Santos, and Santos (1979):

1. Twenty-two percent of alcohol abusers presented as functionally senile due to overdose.

Gomberg (1990):

1. *Aging:* Lower amounts of alcohol produce higher blood levels.

2. Decreases in liver and kidney function make alcohol stay in the body longer.

Hartford and Damorajski (1982):

1. *Sleep:* Reduced REM sleep and reduced stages 3 and 4 sleep (deeper sleep)

2. *Nervous System:* Myopathy, susceptibility to infection, nutritional and vitamin deficiencies

3. *Brain Impairment:* Basal ganglia, hippocampus

---

alcohol, in general, their cognition was greatly improved. Other brain areas such as the basal ganglia, however, affect motor functioning and balance. Other severe side effects of alcoholism are its direct impact on sleep, sexual functioning, and functioning of the stomach and colon.

Myth # 2: Without the alcohol, the older adult will be lonely or depressed.

This myth is often stated as, "Why take away their only pleasure (drinking)?" The truth, of course, is that alcohol is a central nervous system depressant, and that, over time, it causes increased depression and loss of pleasure. Myers et al. (1982) reported in their community sample of elderly alcohol abusers that 22 percent stated that their relationships with others suffered significantly. In addition, those with alcohol problems were significantly less satisfied with their lives than those without drinking problems. Schuckit et al. (1980), in their three-year study of alcohol abuse and treatment, found depression to be more common in their subjects' lives than those without drinking problems. It is precisely because a major hallmark of alcohol abuse in the elderly is that it leaves them lonely and isolated that most authors view socialization and grief work as necessary components to alcohol treatment (Brody, 1982; Kofoed et al., 1987; Sumberg, 1985; Zimberg, 1984). In long-term care, one group of alcoholic patients will come into the facility having no community or family support, saddled with severe debilitating chronic illness and significant cognitive deficits. A second group will come in with significant physical health needs, a lack of community support, but few cognitive problems. This group, often suffering from depression, is more likely to have their alcoholism overlooked (Schukit, 1977).

Myth # 3: Alcohol treatment does not work with the elderly.

This myth is often stated as, "They (alcoholics) are too set in their ways to change." Here, an overview of treatment effectiveness will be reviewed, and, in a later section, discussion of specific aspects of treatment will be explored. Research has repeatedly shown that older alcoholics respond just as well if not better to treatment than do younger adults (Atkinson and Kofoed, 1982; Benshoff and Roberto, 1987; Janik and Dunham, 1983; Schuckit, 1977; Zimberg, 1984). Janik and Dunham reported on the results from 550 alcoholism treatment programs for a total sample of 3,163 older alcoholics (aged 60 and up) and 3,190 younger alcoholics. Self-report and counselor ratings were used to determine follow-up results 180 days after the completion of inpatient treatment. Men, overall, had a poorer treatment outcome than women, and older adults had a significantly better treatment outcome than did middle-aged ones.

Atkinson and Kofoed (1982) and Kofoed et al. (1987) have reported a series of studies in which older alcoholics were more likely to complete treatment successfully and to maintain sobriety for longer periods. In his study of all alcohol treatment programs for the state of Washington, Schuckit (1977) found that while 73 percent of the elderly who started treatment completed it, only 40 percent of younger patients did so. Schuckit did not speculate as to the reason for this. In contrast to younger adults, however, elderly alcohol abusers may experience more directly the ill effects of the alcohol abuse (physical decline, cognitive dysfunction, and social decline). They may, thus, be more motivated or ready to enter treatment.

A final reason why detection is poor relates to the specific deficits associated with alcohol abuse in older adults. The symptoms are often subtle, and the symptoms can be common to other more prevalent syndromes (e.g., dementia, depression). Cognitive deficits in older alcohol abusers may be one of the more common symptoms, and yet is too often perceived as part of a progressive dementia unrelated to alcohol.

Cognitively, the elderly are more vulnerable to the effects of alcohol than a younger person, even with light "social" drinking (Parker and Noble, 1980). Clinicians, however, are often confused because, qualitatively, the cognitive deficits caused by alcohol may be similar to those associated with both normal aging and Alzheimer's dementia. Diagnosis of the etiology of the dementia is important secondary to the differences in prognosis. Studies indicate that approximately 10 percent of alcoholics have severe cognitive deficits (Rains and Ditzler, 1993) while 4 percent of dementia patients have alcohol as the etiology (Larson, Reifler, and Sumi, 1985). In order for a dementia to be associated with alcoholism, both alcohol dependence and dementia criteria must be met, the dementia must persist for at least three weeks after cessation of drinking, and all other causes of dementia must be ruled out. Thus, alcoholic dementia is a diagnosis of exclusion.

Typically, alcohol-related cognitive deficits are subtle, with the maintenance of abilities that contributes to the appearance of intactness in many situations of everyday living. Deficits, however, are seen in complex abilities, such as planning, foresight, and the ability to make appropriate decisions on the basis of available evidence, that result in substantial difficulties in higher adaptive functioning (Goldstein and Levin, 1987). Across studies, however, neuropsychological findings vary with the function assessed and the specific instrument used for assessment (Ryan and Butters, 1986).

Tarter, Van Thiel, and Edwards (1988) suggest that neuropsychological impairment in alcoholics may occur due to both direct and indirect effects. Direct effects result from the toxic effect of alcohol on the brain, while indirect effects may occur secondary to nutritional deficiencies, cerebral trauma or liver disease, and decreased oxygen saturation. Two general models are hypothesized to explain the neuropsychological findings related to age, alcoholism, and performance: (1) "premature aging" model and (2) the "increased vulnerability with age" model (Atkinson and Ganzini, 1994). Findings fitting the "premature aging" model suggest that error scores of alcoholics of any age are equivalent to scores of a nonalcoholic individual 5 to 15 years older. Results of studies fitting the "increased vulnerability with age" model report small, if any, neuropsychological test differences in younger alcoholics while reporting increasingly greater effects in elderly alcoholics. In both models, it is age, rather than duration of alcohol, that seems to determine the degree of alcohol's effect on performance.

Cognitive impairment in recently detoxified alcoholics of all ages is probably multifactorial, representing the effects of chronic alcohol neurotoxicity, withdrawal, depression, and hepatic and metabolic dysfunction. Significant improvements during the first few weeks of sobriety are attributable to all of these factors, although age remains an important predictor of residual deficits three to four weeks after sobriety (Schafer et al., 1991).

TREATMENT OF ALCOHOL ABUSE

Atkinson and Ganzini (1994) suggest three primary goals for substance abuse treatment in the elderly: to stabilize and reduce substance consumption; treat coexisting medical and psychiatric problems; and to set up appropriate social interventions. The common features of traditional outpatient, inpatient, and residential recovery programs for alcoholics are individual and group counseling, introduction to AA, patient education, and family and social services (Marcus, 1993). Abstinence is only the beginning. Specific needs of the elderly that may be incorporated into rehabilitation recovery programs might include discussions about normal physical and cognitive changes that occur with age versus chemical use, how to cope with losses, grief therapy, reminiscence therapy, assertiveness training and familiarization with social support and community resources. The goal is to overcome denial and develop self-awareness, a particular challenge for individuals with cognitive deficits. The family also needs education about the complexity of the problem and their role in supporting recovery. One particularly appealing form of treatment for older adults is group therapy.

Group therapy offers many advantages for the elderly. Groups enable participants to receive positive reinforcement from peers, provide increased opportunity to model both peer and leader behavior, provide an opportunity for social interaction to decrease the common problems of loneliness and isolation, and draw upon the experiences of others with similar problems (Johnson, 1989). Aging issues, such as retirement, physical losses, grief, and isolation, are unique and require special attention in a group context. Specialized AA groups for elderly persons, conducted in rehabilitation hospitals and senior citizens centers, would be particularly beneficial. AA groups need to be tailored to the elderly, with an increased emphasis on socialization and grief counseling. One must question how well the AA model will work with future cohorts of older adults, and whether AA will need to incorporate more of the behavioral and psychosocial knowledge about drinking and alcohol abuse in older adults. The empirical literature on treatment of alcohol abuse in older adults reveals how difficult substance abuse treatment is for all populations and yet how well treatment can work once a patient remains in it.

Few studies have examined the effects of different treatments for the elderly alcoholic. Problems exist both in the lack of a clear definition of alcoholism in the elderly and appropriate measures of outcome. Traditionally, abstinence or reduction in alcohol use has been used; although these are difficult to measure due to inaccuracies in self-report. Liberto, Oslin, and Ruskin (1992) suggest defining outcome in the elderly in terms of improvement in psychosocial function, given the frequently presenting symptoms of social isolation, depression, and loneliness. In rehabilitation, this focus on functional outcome has always been a measure of the amount of services needed and been correlated with the individual's sense of well-being.

Dupree, Broskowski, and Schonfeld (1984) described two treatment efforts. Dupree and his colleagues focused on treating the late onset alcoholics in their Gerontology Alcohol Project, a day-treatment program. Over a two-year period, 406 referrals were made and 153 met the criteria for later-life onset alcohol abuse. Only 48 (31 percent) agreed to treatment, with another one-half dropping out before completing treatment. Thus, 24 patients completed this unique program. Treatment was based on behavioral and self-management techniques. Four treatment modules were developed. The first analyzed the drinking behavior, identifying common antecedents to drinking and developing the behavior chain from general behavior to specific drinking behavior. Module 2 addressed self-management techniques in high-risk situations, such as cues, urges, relapse, depression, anger, and anxiety. Module 3 educated the patients regarding the medical, psychological, statistical, and theoretical aspects of alcohol abuse. The last module focused on general problem solving. Pre- and post-testing revealed the following results. Patients that completed the program learned the material from the different modules. Alcohol consumption was significantly reduced, both in the program and at follow-up. Finally, patients increased the size of their social network. As can be seen from the dropout numbers, only 16 percent of those eligible completed the treatment. Thus, while it is exciting to see such a well-structured program, it is disappointing to see the low rate of compliance with treatment.

Kofoed et al. (1987) tested their hypothesis that elderly alcoholics would respond better to treatment in special elderly peer groups than in mixed age groups and compared the outcomes of two groups of older alcoholics (24 in a mixed-age outpatient group and 25 in an elderly only group). Each group received a 30-day inpatient program followed by the outpatient groups. One year later they compared the two groups. Sixty-eight percent of the patients in the elder only group remained in the treatment program, while only 17 percent of those in the mixed age group did so. A blind retrospective review of records was performed. The treatment group had longer periods of sobriety than did the dropouts. When members of the treatment group relapsed, they were willing to get help and to once again abstain from alcohol. In contrast, members of the dropout group did not get additional help. Though promising results were produced, this sample was a small one and generalizability is limited.

Differences in treatment for the elderly, as compared to a younger age group, might include longer time for detoxification (Douglass, 1984), treatment of multiple medical problems, and modification of medication protocols for withdrawal (Sherose, 1993). Physiologic changes secondary to disability require adaptations such as frequent rest breaks, large print material for education, and minimal writing for those with weakness or arthritis. Treatment should be conducted in a distraction-free environment together with simplifying language and providing repetition of materials in multisensory modalities to minimize the effects of cognitive dysfunction. Outpatient day treatment programs may also provide needed structure to maximize cognitive functioning. In keeping with AA advice, "keep it simple."

ISSUES OF RELAPSE

The few longitudinal studies performed offer encouragement that alcoholism can be treated in the elderly. Nordstrom and Berglund (1987) followed 55 male alcoholics 20 years after their first admission to the hospital. At follow-up, 42 percent still abused alcohol,

38 percent were social drinkers and 20 percent were abstainers. In a three-year follow-up, only 20 percent of active alcoholics seen on a medical unit became abstainers. Once again a self-report methodology was used. The reporting of such a high percentage of alcohol abusers as "social drinkers" runs against widely held beliefs that most alcohol abusers who are drinking cannot control their intake. Whether the findings are reflective of true facts or reflective of response bias these authors have provided some of the only longitudinal data.

Atkinson and Ganzini (1994) investigated hospital readmission for alcohol abuse problems in the Veterans Administration hospital system over a one-year period including 19,000 subjects. Readmission rates for alcohol or drug abuse were approximately 34 percent of the sample. Readmission to the hospital was unrelated to the demographic factors such as sex, age, and race. Unmarried patients, patients with multiple outpatient medical visits, and number of prior inpatient treatment episodes were the best predictors of readmission to the hospital for alcohol problems.

AN INTERDISCIPLINARY APPROACH TO CONFRONTING ALCOHOL ABUSE IN OLDER ADULTS

Geriatric health care settings are loathe to detect and treat the psychosocial aspects of alcohol abuse for a multitude of reasons. A primary concern is cost. Health care settings fear becoming labeled as alcohol rehabilitation centers because treatment can be costly, and reimbursement for this type of treatment with older adults is poor. Geriatrician, physical, occupational therapists, speech language pathologists, nurses, and others are often untrained in alcohol abuse issues with older adults. Nevertheless, it is the distinct impression of most geriatric health care providers that untreated alcohol abuse results in significant morbidity and mortality.

The issue of detecting and treating alcohol abuse was tackled by an interdisciplinary group at our hospital. A physician-led group of nurses, social workers, psychologists, and researchers gathered to address the detection and treatment of alcohol abuse in our facility. One component of this was alcohol abuse in older adults. The goals of the project team were to develop standard screening questions, to develop educational materials and individualized treatment options for alcoholics, and to develop a method of educating families. The CAGE questions and some general follow-up questions were chosen for use in screening.

Treatment options were developed that included attending an Alcoholics Anonymous group that was created at the hospital, psychoeducational presentations, peer counseling from community volunteers, psychotherapy, and educational videos in the patient library. Families were to be encouraged to use the videos and some reading materials.

The group worked together for 18 months before the CAGE became a routine part of the admission process. The slow progress was due mostly to the number of groups that needed to "buy in" to the alcohol treatment effort. This included senior management, service line administrators, the medical records committee, management information systems and the attending physicians. Thus, there are no current outcomes to report. The experience of this project team points out the barriers to be overcome when introducing alcohol abuse treatment in a non "alcohol rehab" program. Still, the need for health care teams to accurately identify and treat older adults alcohol abusers remains an important goal.

Clinical Implications

Alcohol abuse, as was described for depression, can be detected by any member of the interdisciplinary team once the chief symptoms of the syndrome are recognized. In the case of alcohol abuse the symptoms that raise suspicion are general health and social interaction issues. Problems such as unexplained falls or bruises or burns may be recognized by physical and occupational therapy staff who work with patients on a daily basis. Social work staff may discover that the family is no longer engaged with the patient because of an ongoing alcohol abuse problem.

Once recognized, it is vitally important that the mental health practitioner refocus the health care team to treatment of alcohol abuse as a health problem. This includes advocating for an educational approach including the physical, psychological, and social aspects of abuse. A candid discussion or series of discussions should be undertaken with the patient in which the alcohol abuse problem is clearly identified and discussed. Health care professionals are reluctant to assess and treat alcohol abuse, in part because they do not want their program labeled as a substance abuse program. As was described above, however, a limited program of treatment can be pursued. Treatment options, both short (during hospitalization) and long term, should be discussed as well. Here, it is important for the patient to understand the limitations in treatment options that the particular health care setting has. Mental health practitioners, thus, can be leaders in assuring that older adults' alcohol abuse problems are assessed and treated.

Chapter 9

Emerging Areas
in Geriatric Health Care Practice

DETERMINING PATIENT COMPETENCE
AND DECISION-MAKING CAPACITY

The mental health professional's role in determining patient competency is an ever-increasing one, and is increasingly being researched and scrutinized. Competence is a legal concept, and the determination of incompetence can only be established through the judicial system. Mental health professionals, nevertheless, remain intimately involved in these decisions since the courts rely heavily on expert witness evidence (Iris, 1988). This review will be illustrative and not complete (see Moye, 1996 or Grisso, 1994 for more thorough reviews), and will present and critique several research studies of competency. Finally, some guidelines will be presented.

Moye (1996) defined competency as the capacity for self-determination. In terms of civil competency issues, this refers to the determination of self-care or property care capacity (incompetence resulting in a guardian or conservator), and the capacity to consent to medical decisions. Pruchno et al. (1995) stressed that competency is the perception of how well someone can perform when self-care decisions need to be made. State statutes require significant patient deficits in one, two, or three of the following: (1) disorders or disabilities, (2) decision-making/communication disability, and/or (3) functional impairment.

Grisso (1994) provided some important cautions about the determination of incompetence. First, he stated that legal incompetence cannot be determined merely by the presence of a mental disorder. A diagnosis of a neurologic condition does not automatically render one incapable of self-care determination. Disorders must be linked to disabilities. Second, he remarked that legal incompetence is not an all or none status. The question should be incompetent for what? Limited incompetency judgments may become more the norm as opposed to persons losing all competencies. Third, legal incompetence is not to be conceptualized as permanent. Delirium, for instance, may produce an incompetency judgment, but when treated and cured, the patient's self-care determination abilities are regained. Finally, he reminded that there is no single legal definition of incompetence.

Moye (1996) and Grisso (1994) did a nice job of discussing components of competence and its assessment. Grisso identified functional skills (ADLs and IADLs) as one component of competence. Moye noted that there are many functional scales that can be used to measure these abilities. She noted that many of these scales enhance interrater reliability, but that the psychometric properties of many scales are poor. Moye identifies a neuropsychological testing approach as strong in psychometric properties, but both she and Grisso state that a major disadvantage is the relative lack of relationship between test scores and everyday behavior. These conclusions are based, however, on somewhat outdated literature. As presented in an earlier chapter, test scores on standard neuropsychological instruments are highly related to the functional capacities of ADL abilities, medication management, financial abilities, driving, and other IADL skills.

Grisso noted that other components included a causal component. The disability, he noted, must be causally related to the mental disorder. The interactive component of competency refers to how well matched are the individual's abilities with the specific demands of his or her circumstances. Finally, the judgmental component refers to determining when the mismatch between the individuals abilities and his or her demands are sufficiently serious to warrant pursuit of incompetency.

Moye (1996) described other methods used in competency determinations. These included competency guidelines and competency scales. Competency guidelines are the shared beliefs about what must go into competent decision making. These include evidence of choice, appreciation of risks and benefits, understanding of concepts, and rational reasoning for decisions. Competency scales offer the advantage of determining psycholegal definitions of competency and then utilizing normative data. At this time it is our belief that no competency scale has broad enough normative data to be useful in applying the published data to the older adult urban medical patients, who often belong to a minority group, and have less formal education as compared to the control groups used to establish normative data.

Abernathy (1984) reviewed his involvement with a celebrated case in which a patient was judged incompetent because she would not make a decision, nor would she identify risks or benefits of treatment. Abernathy offered two cautions: (1) incompetence must be proved, not just suspected; and (2) good overall cognitive skill would be incompatible with incompetence.

Before we proceed to further discuss methods of competency assessment, and to review several empirical studies, we will focus briefly on the courtroom proceedings that involve guardianship. Iris (1988) conducted a six-month study of guardian decision making by directly observing 141 courtroom proceedings, and by interviewing eleven attorneys. She came to two major conclusions. First, older adults were less likely to appear in court, less likely to contest a petition, and more likely to have a plenary guardian of both estate and person appointed. Second, protests of guardianship with older adults focused on who should become the guardian, and not whether the protection was needed. Keith and Wacker (1993) examined 1,160 court records of older adults' guardianship hearings. The average age of the older adults was 81 years, and while 24 percent were married, only 4 percent lived with their spouse. In all, 75 percent of older adults lived in group facilities. Seventy-nine percent of the guardians were family members. Only 13 percent of wards attended their own hearing, and only 4 percent had their own private attorney represent them. The results of the above studies suggest that guardianship is most often sought for the very frail elderly. Both studies stated clearly that the role of the health care professional was pivotal in the guardianship hearings. Judges relied heavily on the expert testimony of professionals. Experts will experience increasing scrutiny, however, and their recommendations will need to be based upon an empirical foundation. To date, medical decision making has been the only area of competency decisions extensively studied.

EMPIRICAL STUDIES OF MEDICAL DECISION MAKING

Health care researchers agree on the key issues of consent to medical treatments. These include communicating choices, understanding relevant information, appreciation of the situation and consequences, and the ability to manipulate information rationally (Roth, Meisel, and Lidz, 1977; Applebaum and Grisso, 1988). Gutheil and Bursztayn (1986) provided mental health clinicians with some steps to follow in decision making with mentally impaired individuals:

1. Intervene clinically first, and use the court as a last resort.
2. Anticipate thorough documentation, and develop awareness of the competency requirements.
3. Avoid extreme or global judgments, and clearly articulate clinical findings.
4. Enlist family and staff support, and obtain consultation.

Several research efforts will be reviewed and critiqued in the following text.

Fitten and Waite (1990) studied decision making in hospitalized elderly. Three clinical vignettes were developed to assess treatment decision-making capacity. The authors compared 25 medical patients judged to be competent with 25 age- and education-matched normal controls. The mean age of subjects was 68 years, the mean educational level was 12 years, and the mean Mini Mental State Exam was 28. The authors concluded that 28 percent of the patients had significant decisional impairments but that these were not detected by either the Mini Mental State Exam scores or by physician judgment. Using the same vignettes and control group, Fitten, Lusky, and Hamann (1990) investigated treatment decision making in nursing home patients. Veterans Administration nursing home residents, with a mean MMSE score of 22.4 were included. Only 33 percent of these patients demonstrated intact decision making, whereas 77 percent of the patients had been judged competent by their physicians.

The authors concluded that cognitive tests underestimate decisional problems. There is a significant methodological problem with these studies, however. Only 60 percent of the normal controls passed all three vignettes. The solution of the authors was to delete six questions, thereby achieving a 93 percent passing rate. Given this base rate of controls failing it is likely that the questioning of the vignettes was too difficult.

Drane (1984) provided his view that the standard for competent decision making should vary by the dangerousness of the situation. For medical decisions that are not dangerous, awareness and assent are all that is needed. With chronic illness decisions, or more dangerous treatment that has alternative choices, he argued that the patient must understand the risks and outcomes, and make a choice based on that understanding. Finally, for cases where the diagnosis is fairly certain, there is effective treatment, and death is likely due to refusal, there must be the highest degree of understanding demonstrated, and rational decision making evidenced.

Alexander (1988) examined 92 consecutive admissions to a neurobehavioral service in order to assess the prevalence of mental competence. Three steps of competence were assessed: making decisions, passing minimal cognitive criteria, and determining whether the deficit could be compensated for. Forty-seven patients had a single defect in mental competence, and 36 had multiple defects.

Examining the Alexander (1988) and Fitten (Fitten and Waite, 1990; Fitten et al., 1990) studies, together with the standards set by Drane (1984), it is clear that a wide variety of approaches to competence exist. The empirical studies did not investigate what Grisso (1994) highlighted: the need to assess the interaction between a person's abilities, and the demands placed on them. Instead, the empirical studies examined the patients' competencies without assessing the demands of the patients' environments. Drane's standards, in contrast, vary the level of scrutiny used in evaluating competency depending upon the seriousness (i.e., how life threatening) of the medical condition.

Examining the relationship between cognition and competence has been the subject of recent research (Pruchno et al., 1995; Marson et al., 1996; Marson, Cody, Ingram, and Harrell, 1995; Marson, Ingram, Cody, and Harrell, 1995). Pruchno and her colleagues

(1995) examined performance on competency measures in three nursing home units. All subjects had to exceed 15 on their MMSE to be included. Fifty (39 percent of those approached) agreed to participate. Three-quarters were women, the mean level of education was 11 years, and mean age was 86 years. The researchers compared the patients performance on the MMSE, the Hopemont Capacity Assessment Inventory and the Understanding Treatment Disclosure instrument with clinical judgments made by psychologists. Competency scores on a six-point scale, as rated by the psychologists, were highly related to MMSE (r = .70, p<.05), the Hopemont (r = .61, p<.05), and the Understanding Treatment Disclosure recognition task (r = .60, p<.05). Fifty-eight percent of competence variance was explained, and in a discriminant function analysis, there was an 86 percent overall correct classification.

Marson, Ingram, Cody, and Harrell (1995) created two new specialized vignettes in order to focus their research on competency to consent to medical treatment. The vignettes and the questioning take 20 to 25 minutes to administer. Forty-four subjects participated, 15 normal controls and 29 individuals with probable Alzheimer's disease. Subjects had a mean age of 68 years, and a mean educational level of 11 years. Competency was assessed by expert raters across five domains: *Legal Standard 1:* evidence of choice; *Legal Standard 2:* reasonable choice; *Legal Standard 3:* appreciate consequences of choice; *Legal Standard 4:* rational reasons; and *Legal Standard 5:* understanding choice. Interrater reliability was reported at r = .83, p<.05.

There were significant differences between the normal controls and the Alzheimer's disease patients in three of the areas: Legal Standards 3, 4, and 5. All of the Alzheimer's disease patients demonstrated compromise on Legal Standard 5, for instance, whereas all moderately impaired individuals displayed compromise on Legal Standard 4, and 50 percent of the mildly impaired group demonstrated compromised performance on that standard. These last standards are heavily loaded on reasoning and memory tasks, which are hallmark symptoms of even early Alzheimer's disease.

Marson, Cody, Ingram, and Harrell (1995), using the same sample, compared the relationship between a number of neuropsychological test measures with the competency vignette scores for Legal

Standard 4: Rational reasons for treatment choice. Twenty-two neuropsychological measures, covering the domains of language, attention, memory, abstraction and executive functioning were utilized. Eight of the neuropsychological measures correlated significantly with competency scores ranging from r = .44 to r = .60. The best single predictor was the Dementia Rating Scale's one-minute verbal fluency task (naming grocery store items). This accounted for 36 percent of the variance in Alzheimer's patients, and 33 percent of the variance in normals, and correctly classified 82 percent of cases. In multiple regression analyses neither MMSE or any memory measure was a significant predictor of competency scores.

Marson et al. (1996) extended this work by investigating the relationship of the neuropsychological measures with Legal Standards 1, 3, and 5, again using the same sample as the previous two studies. The results were similar to their work on Legal Standard 4. Significant correlations ranged from .44 to .81. Auditory comprehension, verbal fluency, confrontation naming and conceptualization were the best predictors of standards 1, 3, and 5 respectively. Overall, correct classifications ranged from 91 to 98 percent. The work of Marson and his colleagues is creative and impressive research. The authors utilize a new competency assessment tool, and correlated it with performance-based cognitive measures. The weaknesses of the research must be noted as well, however. These include a small sample, and a patient population limited to only those with Alzheimer's disease.

LIMITATIONS IN COMPETENCY ASSESSMENT RESEARCH

While the creation of face-valid vignettes may appear to be an excellent solution to the assessment of competent decision making, there are a number of limitations to this approach. The major weaknesses of this approach are as follows: (1) A set of interview questions following a vignette loads heavily on attentional and organizational skills. Immediate recall of stories—on cognitive testing for instance—may be less important than the rate of forgetting. Similarly, using an interview that taps only into immediate recall of vignette material may underemphasize the role of memory in assessments; (2) Poor normative data. Competency assessments have a very small and unrepresentative normative base. To use these instruments, and the available normative data in clinical situations with urban older adult medical patients, for example, may lead to the incorrect classification of incompetence in independent functioning individuals. This is a corollary to the neuropsychological test results reported in an earlier chapter. Normative data must be gathered on samples that approximate one's patient population before the scale should be used clinically. (3) Extreme limitations in generalizability. The limits of generalizability echo the concerns about normative data. The available data cannot, at present, be generalized to many clinical situations. (4) The neglected role of memory in competency assessment. There are few delayed recall or recognition paradigms for competency assessments, despite the fact that delayed recall represents the best assessment of memory. It makes no sense to us, that even though memory functioning is the hallmark symptom of dementia, it plays a minimal role in competency assessments. The ability to recall risks and benefits, the rationale used for making a decision, and the possible outcomes of treatment are core components of competent decision making; and (5) No consideration of awareness of deficit. Awareness of deficit must exist if a patient is able to utilize effective compensatory strategies. The assessment of awareness and compensation should then play an integral role in the competency assessment process. Awareness of deficit about the patient's dementia can also help assess the patient's level of awareness for making a certain medical decision, or his or her level of awareness of what skills are required to continue living alone.

The assessment of competency is a growing role of mental health practitioners in geriatric health care settings. Expanded clinical models of assessment and clinical research will continue to grow in this area. It is our belief that until some of the major limitations of vignette approaches are addressed the following guidelines can be used for competency assessment. Measure function in multiple domains: physical and self-care, cognitive awareness of deficit, and compensation and competency instrument assessments. Consider the tasks or judgments required for the patient to make, and integrate these into the competency decisions. If for example, a clinician is judging the capabilities of a demented person to live independently, the awareness of deficit, cognitive, and IADL data should be tied together. One final reminder: Do not rely solely on competency assessment instruments, particularly if the patient is less educated, or significantly older than the normative sample. Competency evaluation methods will continue to grow and improve, and thereby improve the services offered to older adults in health care settings.

A Technical Advisory Group was assembled by the Veteran's Administration in 1996 in order to improve geropsychological practice. As their first task, this group addressed the issue of competency assessment in older adults. The following outline represents their conclusions:

Step 1:   Clarify the referral. Determine the reasonableness of the request and obtain the specific question (i.e., competent for what).

Step 2:   Obtain informed consent, arrange for medical, social, psychiatric, and legal data to be available for review. Arrange to interview the patient and key informants.

Step 3:   Assess cognition. Assess all cognitive domains. Select tests which are reliable and valid and for which there are norms approximating the age and educational background of the patient. Attend to ecological validity by selecting tests which have empirical support in predicting function. Assess patient's awareness of cognitive deficits.

Step 4:   Clarify which specific capacities are in question (i.e., finances, driving, cooking, etc.). Use tests that measure actual performance on functional ability tasks rather than rely on self or informant report.

Step 5:   Attend to the impact of mental health status on cognitive and functional performance, especially depression and anxiety. Gather mental health status data from multiple sources, including family and other professionals.

Step 6:   Write a report documenting the reason for referral, the methods utilized, the findings of the assessment, the specific response to the referral question, and other recommendations. Provide direct feedback to the patient.

Following these six steps will help ensure that a thorough and high-quality assessment has been completed.

TREATMENT OF PAIN AND ANXIETY

Anxiety is a common condition in older adults, and one that becomes more central in the midst of physical health problems and pain. Himmelfarb and Murrell (1984) investigated the prevalence of anxiety in community-dwelling elderly in Kentucky. Thirteen hundred women and 713 men were interviewed for this epidemiological study, and 21 percent of women, and 17 percent of men reported high levels of anxiety on the 20-item State-Trait Anxiety Inventory. Anxiety was highest for those between age 75 and 79 as compared to those younger and older. Only 4 percent of the respondents reported seeking help for anxiety, but the anxious group had a higher level of physician visits than did the nonanxious group. The strongest correlate of anxiety, however, was physical health symptoms ($r = .60$) as measured by the presence of diseases and the respondent's perception of his/her health. These data suggest then that anxiety is closely tied to illness and to pain. Barbee and McLaulin (1990) posited that anxiety results from a loss of personal control over critical events in one's internal and external environment. Hospitalization, illness, and disability can bring powerful feelings of loss of control.

Studies of pain in older adults residing in both community and institutional settings reported that pain is a frequent experience in this population (Lavsky-Shulan et al., 1985; Ferrell, Ferrell, and Osterweil, 1990). In a study of over 3,000 Iowans, lower back pain was present in 24 percent of women, and 18 percent of men. Pain was associated with several important functional and health conditions including decreased sleep (21 percent), analgesic medication use (50 percent), and decreased household chores and bending. Over a quarter of those reporting pain problems were hospitalized at least once due to the pain.

Ferrell, Ferrell, and Osterweil (1990) investigated pain in 97 nursing home patients. The average age of the subjects was 89 years and 85 percent were women. Patients were interviewed, and medical records were investigated to determine the prevalence of pain complaints. Whereas 71 percent of the sample had at least one pain complaint, 34 percent of pain complainers had constant pain. There was a significant relationship between pain and attendance in activities ($r = .50$), but no relation between pain and depression, cognition, and ADL abilities. Clearly, then, pain is a common experience in older adults in health care settings.

The influence of psychological factors on pain in older adults has only been investigated for 10 to 15 years. We produced some of the earliest data on this topic when we investigated the experience of pain in those with knee osteoarthritis (Lichtenberg, Skehan, and Swensen, 1984; Lichtenberg, Swensen, and Skehan, 1986). In the first study 40 older adults were given the McGill Pain Questionnaire, the Hypochondriacal and Depression scales from the MMPI, and the Social Readjustment Rating Scale. The severity of the degenerative disease was rated on a five-point scale by a rheumatologist blind to the pain ratings. Hypochondriasis scores were significantly correlated with pain ($r = .61$, $p<.001$), whereas arthritic severity was not ($r = .00$). In the second study a larger sample was recruited ($n = 70$), and several domains of coping and activity levels were included.

Multiple regression was utilized to determine the best predictors of pain. Arthritic severity was entered first, and was a significant predictor of pain, accounting for 13 percent of pain variance. The psychological variables accounted for an additional 41 percent of variance. Hypochondriasis held the strongest correlation to pain ($r = .60$, $p <.001$), but several other variables including health promotive and destructive behaviors, daily hassles, and social activity also were significantly related to perceived pain. The results of these studies suggest that psychological factors may play a significant role in the experience of pain in older adults.

Casten et al. (1995) recently investigated the relationship of pain and anxiety in older adults. They posited three hypotheses that might account for the relationship between pain and anxiety: (1) *the muscle tension hypothesis:* anxious people have more muscle tension causing muscle tightening which then leads to increased pain; (2) *the arousal hypothesis:* increased arousal with anxiety may lead to decreased pain tolerance; and (3) *the complainer hypothesis:* although anxiety may not alter the perception of pain, anxious individuals are more likely to complain of pain. The authors then studied the experience of pain, anxiety, and depression in 365 congregate apartment, and 114 nursing home dwellers. Pain intensity was measured by a six-item questionnaire developed by one of the authors, and number of pain complaints was assessed by questions regarding 12 areas of the body. Anxiety and depression were measured by a 35-item checklist and the Profile of Mood States. The results indicated that there was a high comorbidity of anxiety and depression. Anxiety was significantly related to pain intensity ($r = .26$, $p < .001$), and to pain complaints ($r = .34$, $p < .001$).

While Casten et al. (1995) were the first to specifically study anxiety and pain, their study had a number of limitations. First, their sample, although having a mean age of 83 years, was composed of all white respondents, limiting the generalizability of these findings to minority elderly. Second, the authors did not attempt to test the different hypotheses about the reasons for the anxiety-pain linkage, thereby limiting any implications for treatment.

Understanding the specific symptoms of anxiety that are related to chronic pain is critical to understanding better the anxiety-pain link. Research in this area was first done with a younger sample (DeGood, Buckelew, and Tait, 1985), and later replicated with an older sample (Parmelee, Kleban, and Katz, in press). DeGood, Buckelew, and Tait (1985) pointed out that anxiety can be broken into cognitive symptoms (e.g., fears, phobias, obsessions), and into somatic symptoms (e.g., increased pulse, gastrointestinal (GI) upset). These authors compared a group of college students with a group of patients who experienced chronic pain (back, hip, and leg) for over two years, and a group of 30 health care professionals on the Cognitive-Somatic-Anxiety Questionnaire. The results indicated two things: (1) pain patients, despite experiencing a disrupted life due to pain, reported less anxiety overall than the other groups; and (2) the pattern of anxiety symptoms endorsed were different for chronic pain patients versus college students and health care professionals. The pain patients endorsed higher levels of somatic anxiety symptoms as opposed to cognitive symptoms of anxiety. The other groups, in contrast, reported higher levels of cognitive anxiety symptoms as opposed to somatic anxiety symptoms. These authors concluded that pain patients were poorly attuned to emotional responses.

Parmelee, Kleban, and Katz (in press) studied the structure of the anxiety-pain relationship in older adults. Their sample of 690 respondents were evaluated for pain, anxiety, depression, medical burden, and ADL skills. Symptoms of pain and anxiety were analyzed and three factors resulted including a depressed mood factor, a somatic symptom factor, and a psychic anxiety factor. The strongest relationship of the factors to pain was between somatic symptoms and pain, similar to the study of DeGood, Buckelew, and Tait (1985). Even when physical health and functional abilities were controlled for, the relationship between somatic symptoms of anxiety and pain remained strong. Depression, interestingly, served as a moderator variable, in that for those with minor depression, psychic anxiety was the best predictor of pain, whereas somatic anxiety was the best predictor of pain in those with a major depression. The authors concluded that somatic symptoms of affective distress are central to the experience of pain. These data may lend support to the arousal hypothesis of the etiology of the pain-anxiety link, and hopefully will lead to direct investigation of that and the other hypotheses being directly tested.

Oberle et al. (1990) studied the experience of anxiety and acute pain in a longitudinal fashion. They utilized 41 surgery patients over the age of 65 years, and 249 patients less than age 65 in a study of pain up to three days after surgery. Pre-op anxiety was unrelated to post-op pain, and at day two after surgery there was no difference between pain reports in the younger and older group. Post-op anxiety, however, was significantly related to post-op pain in both groups for day two ($r = .42$, $p < .05$), and for day three ($r = .42$, $p < .05$). The experience of acute surgical pain was thus similar between younger and older adults, and the experience of anxiety in conjunction with the pain (post-op) produced increased report of pain in older adults.

The data, although limited in terms of volume, are directly applicable to geriatric health care settings. First, there will be a large number of older adults experiencing acute and/or chronic pain in the health care setting. Second, there will be a high comorbidity between pain complaints and anxiety (and depression). Third, there will be a large clinical need for the mental health professional to help the patients' cope with the pain and not over rely on medication. Thus, clinicians need a framework for understanding how to work with pain in older adults.

The gate control theory of pain (Melzack and Wall, 1965) emphasized that sensory inputs, thoughts, and emotions can all affect how much pain is gated to the spinal cord. This created a clear theoretical rationale for psychologists to become treatment providers with chronic pain patients. Dale and DeGood (in press) emphasized, however, that patients with chronic pain must be prepared for a psychological consultation. This includes three elements: (1) Clear communication from the physician to the patient about why psychological consultation is sought. Patients may feel that the physician is merely frustrated with the patient, and trying to shuttle the patient off to the psychologist. The referring physician must be active in explaining the roles of the psychologist in treating pain; (2) Defuse the "sanity hearing" and "organic vs. functional" myths. The myth that pain is experienced due to mental illness, or to being not real, and all in the patient's head must be defused. Sharing the gate theory of pain with the patient can be helpful; (3) Shaping adaptive beliefs. Discussing methods of promoting less pain and better health such as exercise, weight control, and the use of non-narcotic medication.

The assessment of the pain patient can encompass several areas. Dale and DeGood (in press) emphasize the importance of assessing pain-related contingencies (gains and losses that accompany the pain). In addition, assessing patient's beliefs about treatment and the setting of realistic goals is vital before embarking upon treatment.

Treatment in the hospitalized geriatric patient is likely to be limited to relaxation and imagery, and possibly hypnosis and/or biofeedback. Guided deep breathing and imagery can be quite useful in calming down anxious, hurting patients, and provide them with a sense of relief. It is during this time that discussing the other useful health behaviors is suggested. There are no data on the treatment of pain in older adults hospitalized for medical or rehabilitation problems. This would be a fruitful area of research. Nevertheless, pain and anxiety syndromes are a frequent source of difficulty for the patient and a source of referral for the mental health practitioner.

PRACTICE MANAGEMENT ISSUES
FOR THE HEALTH CARE PROVIDER

Clinicians must serve as educators to health care administrators in terms of current billing and revenue practices. This section will focus on psychology practices within health care settings, with an emphasis on Medicare. There are many arrangements that psychologists can have with hospitals. The psychologists may be staff members, they may have a contractual arrangement with the hospital that allows them to be the sole providers of service without being on staff, and/or they may receive a small percentage of salary from the hospital for administrative duties, and receive the rest of their salary based on billings and collections. Psychologists may have their own department, or be services within medical departments such as Psychiatry, Rehabilitation, or Neurology. No matter what the practice arrangement is, psychologists must familiarize themselves with current Medicare regulations, billing, and reimbursement practices.

Psychologists applying to be Medicare providers will have the option of choosing a designation as either an independent practitioner or a clinical psychologist. Independent practitioners are reimbursed under Medicare only for outpatient diagnostic services, and only when there is a physician referral (American Psychological Association, 1994). Qualified clinical psychologists are eligible for reimbursement from Medicare for both therapy and diagnostic services in both inpatient and outpatient settings. In addition, physician referral is not a requirement for reimbursement to clinical psychologists.

In 1992 the Health Care Financing Administration implemented a system of determining charges that takes into account practice costs, time, and work. At the time of this writing, this system addressed only diagnostic services for psychologists and not therapy services. Patients should be billed at a regular rate, although psychologists can only collect Medicare's approved charge. Psychology charges, like physician charges, can be reimbursed independently from what the hospital collects from Medicare for other aspects of hospital care. Medicare Part A refers to hospital insurance benefits, and covers institutional services for inpatients. Medicare Part B refers to medical insurance benefits and covers inpatient and outpatient services of physicians, psychologists, and some other nonphysician providers.

Services are billed for under procedure codes. The following procedure codes are available for psychologists to bill under. These five-digit numerical codes are obtained from the *Physician's Current Procedural Terminology (CPT)* (1995). The most often used codes are the following:

- 90801: includes diagnostic interview examination including history, mental status and disposition. In 1997 psychotherapy codes for individual treatment became more detailed, and because of the number of codes involved these are not reviewed here.
- 96100: is a psychological testing code which includes assessment of personality, psychopathology, and/or intellectual abilities and results in a written report.
- 96115: refers to a neurobehavioral status exam which includes clinical assessment of thinking, reasoning, judgement, memory, etc.
- 96117: refers to a neuropsychological testing battery.

Providing clinical service does not ensure that the service is reimbursable. Medicare requires that the service be medically necessary. If services are provided that are not medically necessary Medicare may refuse to reimburse for the service. Medical necessity is not always clearly defined. In performing evaluations to determine mental competency (as ordered by the court for example), Medicare will not reimburse this service. Performing an evaluation to determine a patient's capability to return to living alone, however, though it might lead to a recommendation of guardianship, is reimbursable. Psychologists are thus urged to educate themselves as to current professional standards regarding medically necessary services.

Chapter 10

Mental Health Practitioners' Survival of Health Care Changes

BETTER UTILIZATION OF INTERDISICIPLINARY TEAM MEMBERS

Mental health practitioners will need to better understand the health care model they work in, better articulate the linkage between their services and outcome data, and better shape the referral process, if they are to survive the influx of managed care, downsizing, and cost reduction. Much of what has been written in the previous chapters provides ammunition for the inclusion of assessment and intervention clinical protocols for use in geriatric health care settings. To effectively utilize this information, however, mental health clinicians will need to better understand how their training may clash with the values of the medical model, still the predominant model of health care delivery in hospital systems. After these model differences are explored, mental health practitioners will be shown one way to alter their own traditional behaviors and to improve referral patterns.

Brown and Zimberg (1982) articulated the professional value differences found in those health practitioners who focused mainly on medical practices with those professionals who focused mainly on mental health practices. Value differences, they argued, were at the basis of many conflicts between practitioners with different orientations. In medical practice, one approaches a problem by ruling out disease, whereas mental health practice rules in all aspects of emotional functioning. Medical practice is action-oriented, and mental health treatment is relatively slower. Medical practitioners act in an executive capacity, assuming responsibility for all decisions. In contrast, mental health practitioners seek a partnership with their patients and spend time creating a trusting relationship. Medical schools' focus on the body makes psychological processes seem superficial. Finally, affect is managed differently by the different practitioners. Medical practice requires that affect be isolated and kept from interfering with a procedure, whereas in mental health practice, affect is utilized in treatment.

Qualls and Czirr (1988) extended the work of Brown and Zimberg by describing the continuum of group processes that treatment teams contend with. Time spent by the team on making treatment decisions can range from quick to long, and to using only factual data (i.e., lab values) to process issues (i.e., compensatory skills). Decision-making models range from those where one team member makes all of the primary decisions to a group consensus. Finally, the importance of teamwork varies considerably between health care teams ranging from total autonomy to interdisciplinary practice. Qualls and Czirr encourage team members to learn about the practice of other disciplines.

Mental health practitioners must inform themselves about the work of the attending physician. This is necessary to better understand how the medical model of training (as highlighted by Brown and Zimberg, 1982; and Qualls and Czirr, 1988) shapes a physician's treatment planning and decision making. We recommend that the mental health practitioner accompany the attending physicians on rounds at least two to three times weekly. By attending rounds the mental health practitioner familiarizes himself with the general and emergency medical issues confronted by that attending physician. This will enable the mental health practitioner to better appreciate what the demands are on the physician for patient care, and what the demands are on the patient for recovery. Issues such as treatment compliance and the experience of acute and chronic pain, for example, are better understood. In addition, mental health issues will spontaneously arise, and the mental health practitioner can help inform physicians on these issues, thereby demonstrating usefulness in achieving good patient outcomes. In our experience, it is precisely issues of depression, anxiety, or fear that the medical model has left physicians feeling ill prepared, and where they appreciate the mental health involvement. Many attending physicians are surprised and impressed, for example, to the extent that patients share their innermost concerns to mental health professionals during the hospital stay. The ability to detect problems of dementia and depression, hidden to the physician, allow mental health practitioners to take the lead in treatment planning.

It is incumbent upon mental health practitioners to learn about all other members of the interdisciplinary team, not just the physicians. This includes observing and interacting with physical and occupational therapists, speech pathologists, and nurses. The key to successful relations with other team members is to make the mental health problems pertinent to the other team member's work. After completing an assessment of cognition that shows a patient has significant problems, for example, we seek out staff that are working with that patient and ask for their input. Open-ended questions are the best way to invite input. How is the patient doing in therapy? Did you notice any signs of confusion? How does our finding of cognitive decline fit with what you've observed? are a few of the questions that can be routinely used to encourage dialogue. In team conferences, mental health practitioners can foster better rapport with other allied health staff by simply asking for input. After occupational and physical therapists report on certain patients, for example, we routinely ask, did you notice signs of depression? or how well did she retain newly taught information? In this way the mental health practitioner can not only improve relations, but also improve their assessment by integrating the observations of others.

Team conflict is frequently detrimental to the mental health practitioner. This need not be the case. Too often, mental health and other allied health staff act as if they are competing to find the single right answer. A therapist's observation that directions are routinely forgotten should not be ignored if the mental health practitioner previously reported no signs of memory problems. Yet it has been observed that this is a mistake often made by mental health practitioners. Instead, further observation, cotreatment, and perhaps further assessment is warranted. Conflicts are inevitable, however, on interdisciplinary teams, but they must be used to improve care and facilitate relations among staff.

Four steps to conflict resolution are encouraged. First, separate the person from the problem. It is important not to let personal animosities become a central focus of a professional conflict. Focus on the problem, rather than personality. To better concentrate on the issue at hand, spend time determining step two: focus on goals, not on methodology. Too often team members argue over methods (i.e., the means of doing something, the "how to") before they have clarified the desired outcome. That is, determine what are the goals for the patient—not just whose treatment plan is to be used. Too often conflicts are heightened when people become entrenched in an expressed viewpoint and, consequently, they lose sight of the treatment goals. Focusing on goals rather than positions is a second step toward deescalating the emotional tug of war between team members. Third, generate alternative methods of reaching the desired goal(s). Brainstorming can elicit new and creative solutions. The final step is to choose a solution based upon some objective standard. This solution should be monitored and assessed as to its utility.

SHAPING REFERRALS IN HEALTH CARE SETTINGS

Improving one's knowledge of medical practices, and ensuring good relations with other interdisciplinary team members, can help mental health practitioners achieve good position to shape the referrals they receive. We have three main observations of current health care trends: (1) Mental health assessments and treatments must be brief; (2) Mental health practice must be tied to health outcomes; and (3) Mental health procedures must have a clear purpose (i.e., specific referral question). Lengths of stays within hospital settings are on the decline, and therefore inpatient work must be briefer. Health care services are more frequently scrutinized, and therefore, mental health services must be targeted and clearly related to outcome. A decision tree created in conjunction with an attending physician in order to improve referral patterns to us is described in the following text.

The issues that led to the decision tree creation were diverse. First, we demonstrated that problems of cognitive decline, which were of critical importance to some patient's discharge planning, were routinely missed on the physician's history and physical examination. This led to several last-minute referrals, and to a delay in patient discharges. It was discovered that patients who expressed the goal to return to living alone were unable to do so because of lack of therapy progress secondary to dementia. By the time this was realized, however, the patient's discharge had to be postponed. Second, the outcome of assessment was clearly delineated. For example, it was demonstrated through empirical data that cognition was the strongest predictor of discharge in patients that lived alone prior to admission to the hospital. Finally, the physician was convinced to use simple, brief, standardized instruments and quantitative scoring to help detect cognitive problems. A set of questions then helped guide the decision-making process. This ultimately led to a decision tree.

Cognition (thinking skills) as we have demonstrated, plays a major role in determining the capacities of older adults. Health care providers are often confronted with having to make recommendations about the ways that a particular patient's cognitive functioning and impairment will limit their instrumental activities of daily living (e.g., decision making, driving, independent living). Medically ill older adults present to hospitals with a higher prevalence of cognitive impairment than is found in the community. For example, in the Hanks and Lichtenberg (1996) study reviewed earlier, whereas only 15 percent of older adults ages 60 to 79 in the community suffer from dementia, over 40 percent of the hospitalized sample ages 60 to 79 suffered from cognitive impairment.

Because they are not familiar with utilizing formal assessment instruments for cognition, many medical and nursing personnel do not recognize the presence of the cognitive disorders in their patients. This makes sense when one considers that many patients are admitted to health care settings for only "medical" reasons, such as a broken hip, a knee replacement, or an acute illness or surgery. It is only when there is a focus on broad health outcomes, and an understanding of the relationship between cognition and capacity that cognitive abilities become an area of interest for medical and nursing personnel. In the past, medical rehabilitation and geriatric evaluation units referred all patients for screening. With cost-containment changes becoming rampant in health care, a specific rationale for referrals is needed. Figure 10.1 is a decision tree created to provide guidelines to

FIGURE 10.1. Decision Tree for Neuropsychology Referral

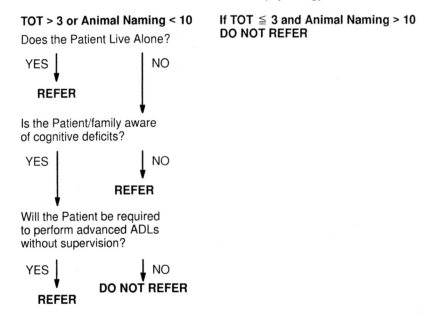

TOT > 3 or Animal Naming < 10

Does the Patient Live Alone?

YES ↓ | NO

REFER

Is the Patient/family aware
of cognitive deficits?

YES | ↓ NO

REFER

Will the Patient be required
to perform advanced ADLs
without supervision?

YES ↓   ↓ NO

REFER   **DO NOT REFER**

**If TOT ≤ 3 and Animal Naming > 10
DO NOT REFER**

A legitimate option is not to refer for Neuropsychology evaluation. This will typically occur when there is no evidence of cognitive deficits, or there is evidence of moderate to severe cognitive deficits, and the family caregiver is aware of these deficits and is or will be providing 24-hour supervision.

primary care and medical rehabilitation physicians as to when to refer patients for cognitive or neuropsychological assessment.

The decision tree assesses three components: basic cognition, patient and family awareness of cognitive problems, and level of patient independence. Basic cognition is assessed by two tests: the Temporal Orientation Test (TOT) and the Animal Naming Test (Benton et al. 1994). Benton and his colleagues provided normative data regarding the TOT and, in their sample of 162 older adults ages 65 to 85, no more than 6 percent of cognitively unimpaired older adults scored in the impaired range on the test. Morris et al. (1989) provided norms for age and education for another simple test to use as a screen for cognition, the Animal Naming task. Although Morris's norms do show changes in animal naming with age, we decided that using a single cutoff score would be easier for referral sources.

If the patient fails one of the screening exams, a patient's living situation is assessed. Patients living alone are then referred for an evaluation. If the patient does not live alone, then the patient and family awareness of a cognitive impairment is assessed before a consultation is sought. If both the patient and family are well aware of the problem, a cognitive evaluation may not be called for. Often, however, patients and families are not aware of these problems. Finally, the level of caregiver support is assessed. If the patient is expected to perform unsupervised instrumental activities of daily living once he or she returns home, the patient is referred for an evaluation. This decision tree helps to remove referrals on cognitively unimpaired patients, and to eliminate referrals on patients who are moderately to severely impaired cognitively who will be receiving 24-hour caregiver support upon discharge. Two case examples are presented to demonstrate the usefulness of this screening procedure across many levels of age and education.

Case #1

Mr. M was a 68-year-old, African-American, retired custodial worker who tripped, fell, and broke his right hip while at home. He had completed only seven years of education. He lived alone at the time of the fall, and upon admission to the medical rehabilitation unit underwent a medical history and physical examination from the attending physician who used the decision tree. Although Mr. M scored in the unimpaired range on the Temporal Orientation Test, because he lived alone the Animal Naming task was given. Mr. M could not name a single animal. He was referred for an assessment of his cognitive abilities. Test results later confirmed by both CT and MRI scans found severe diffuse cerebral dysfunction. He and his family were educated about his condition, and he was later discharged to his daughter's home.

Case #2

Mrs. H was an 86-year-old, white, retired public relations executive who slipped on the ice and fractured her right ankle. Mrs. H, who completed 18 years of education, was extremely conversational and although she was well oriented, the animal naming task was given to her because she lived alone. She obtained a score of 6 on the task and was referred for an evaluation. Her cognitive evaluation revealed significant memory, naming, and mental flexibility deficits that were consistent with a progressive dementia. A family meeting was held, and Mrs. H entered an assisted living setting upon discharge.

RECOGNIZING OPPORTUNITY IN HEALTH SYSTEMS

The changes in health care settings promote anxiety and dread, but also provide opportunity. We have observed that health care no longer takes place in a hospital; health services are delivered in a "health care system." Continuum of care is a popular buzzword in newly organized and configured health systems. That is, hospitals are joining together, or if previously affiliated are now better integrating their services, in order to provide patients with all of their needed health services. Thus, large organizations are now attempting to provide primary care, hospital care, home health care, rehabilitation, and long-term care in an integrated fashion. Conceptually, this model is exciting for mental health practitioners since it could conceivably be possible for practitioners to better track and work with their patients across a variety of settings. Translating conceptual opportunity into real benefits depends upon an openness to new relationships, and an openness to practicing in diverse settings.

Outpatient geriatric health and nursing home care represent two of the best settings in which mental health practitioners can become involved. Developing a working partnership with the staff physicians and nurses in outpatient offices can be centered around the issues of comorbidity of physical and mental health problems, with a focus on outcomes: improved symptomatology in patients, and reduced usage of more expensive health care resources. The mental health practitioner will need, in this setting, to become comfortable with rapidly establishing rapport, and narrowing evaluation to answer the one or two specific referral concerns or questions. Common referral questions include a cognitive evaluation to help diagnose dementia, and psychological evaluations to diagnose and treat affective anxiety, pain, and psychotic disorders. Brief evaluations followed by timely notes with practical recommendations may provide the referral source with the needed information.

Nursing homes are changing as drastically as any health care entity in America. Lichtenberg (1994) addresses mental health practice in long-term care facilities in which a comprehensive approach to psychological services was offered. *A Guide to Psychological Practice in Geriatric Long-Term Care* highlights that patients from mental health facilities were increasingly finding their ways to nursing homes, even when they had active psychotic symptoms. Since that book was written, health care systems have designated nursing homes as sites for medical rehabilitation treatment as well. Indeed, subacute rehabilitation programs are growing exponentially in nursing homes. These dramatic changes in settings for health care delivery are fueled by cost issues. The daily charge (per diem) of care is significantly lower in a nursing home than in a hospital. Thus, to reduce costs, especially cost per discharge, health care systems are acquiring nursing homes and using them for medical rehabilitation programs.

Nursing home practice can either be a very rewarding or a very frustrating endeavor for mental health practitioners. Lichtenberg (1994) reviewed the unique issues of interdisciplinary teams in nursing homes, the wide variety of clinical problems from depression to sexual disturbance, and the need for more mental health workers to assist with patient problems. Readers are encouraged to use that resource when embarking upon work in nursing homes. One way to begin nursing home work is to become involved in the subacute rehabilitation program. Typically these programs consist of older adult patients. The profile of the patients in the subacute programs we have serviced were similar to the ones described earlier for our acute medical rehabilitation inpatients. Thus the issues of high comorbid mental and physical health problems are evident along with the need for assessment, discharge recommendations, and treatments. Home health care and assisted living may represent the programs where future opportunities lie for mental health practitioners. Billing for services in outpatient health or nursing homes can be accomplished through the use of Medicare Part B (see Chapter 9 on emerging trends).

SUMMARY

This chapter ties together the information preceding it and encourages new growth for mental health practitioners in health care settings. Using data on comorbidity and effect of mental health variables on health outcomes, for example, can be useful in advocating mental health services. Good communication with medical and other staff is necessary to make these services a reality. It is also essential to provide the tools for these staff to detect mental health problems. Changes in health care systems will undoubtedly impact mental health practitioners. Ideas concerning methods to target new venues for service delivery are discussed as examples of new partnerships that mental health practitioners can form with medical staff across the continuum of care. Improving the models of mental health practice in health care settings will undoubtedly rest upon empirical evidence of outcomes, brief and cost-effective models of service, and a good understanding of medical health care systems.

References

Introduction

Brody, E.M., Kleban, M.H., and Moles, E.B. (1983). What older people do about their day to day mental and physical health symptoms. *Journal of the American Geriatrics Society, 31*, 489-498.

Hertz, P. (1989). *Quality Improvement Training Manual.* Miami, FL: The Paul Hertz Group.

Hirshorn, B.A. (1993). *An Assessment of the Formal Health and Social Support Needs of Central City Detroit's Older Population.* Report to the Hannan Foundation. Detroit, MI:

Lichtenberg, P.A. (1994). *A Guide to Psychological Practice in Geriatric Long-Term Care.* Binghamton, NY: The Haworth Press.

Lichtenberg, P.A., Gibbons, T.A., Nanna, M.J., and Blumenthal F. (1993). The effects of age and gender on the prevalence and detection of alcohol abuse in elderly medical inpatients. *Clinical Gerontologist, 13(3),* 17-27.

Lichtenberg, P.A., and Rosenthal, M. (1994). Characteristics of geriatric rehabilitation programs: A survey of practitioners. *Rehabilitation Psychology, 39,* 277-281.

Rapp, S.R., Parisi, S.A., and Walsh, D.A. (1988). Psychological dysfunction and physical health among elderly medical inpatients. *Journal of Consulting and Clinical Psychology, 56,* 851-855.

Schuckit, M.A., Atkinson, J.H., Miller, P.L., and Berman, J. (1980). A three-year follow-up of elderly alcoholics. *Journal of Clinical Psychiatry, 41,* 412-416.

Chapter 1

Blazer, D., Hughes, D., and George, L. (1987). The epidemiology of depression in an elderly community population. *The Gerontologist, 27,* 281-287.

Charlson, M.E., Pompei, P., Ales, K.L., and MacKenzie, C.R. (1987). A new method of classifying prognostic comorbidity in longitudinal studies: Development and validation. *Journal of Chronic Diseases, 40,* 373-383.

Evans, D.A., Funkenstein, H., Albert, M.S., Scherr, P.A., Cook, N.R., Chown, M.J., Hebert, L.F., Hennekens, C.H., and Taylor, J.O. (1989). Prevalence of Alzheimer's disease in a community population of older persons. *Journal of the American Medical Association, 262,* 2551-2556.

Hanks, R.A., and Lichtenberg, P.A. (1996). Physical, psychological and social outcomes in geriatric rehabilitation patients. *Archives of Physical Medicine and Rehabilitation, 77,* 783-792.

Lichtenberg, P.A., Ross, T.P., Millis, S.R., and Manning, C.A. (1995). The relationship of depression and cognition in older adults: A cross-validation study. *Journal of Gerontology: Psychological Sciences, 50B*, P25-P32.

Mattis, S. (1988). *dementia Rating Scale: Professional Manual.* Odessa, FL: Psychological Assessment Resources.

Wechsler, D. (1987). *The Wechsler Memory Scale–Revised.* New York: Psychological Corporation.

Welis, C.E. (1979). Pseudodementia. *American Journal of Psychiatry, 136*, 895-900.

Yesavage, J., Brink, T., Rose, T., Lum, O., Huang, V., Adez, M., and Leirer, V. (1983). Development and validation of a Geriatric Depression Screening Scale: A preliminary report. *Journal of Psychiatric Research, 17*, 37-49.

Chapter 2

Anderson, S., and Tranel, D. (1989). Awareness of disease states following cerebral infarction, dementia, and head trauma: Standardized assessment. *The Clinical Neuropsychologist, 3*, 327-339.

Babinski, M.J. (1914). Contribution a l'etude des troubles mentax dans l'hemiplegie organique cerebrale (Anosognosie). *Revue Neuroligique, 12*, 845-848.

Bergmann, K., Proctor, S., and Prudham, D. (1979). Symptom profiles in hospital and community resident elderly persons with dementia. In F. Hoffmeister and C. Muller (Eds.), *Brain Function in Old Age* (pp. 139-163). Berlin: Springer-Verlag.

Caron, J. (1996). *The Role of Cognition and Awareness of Deficit in Predicting ADL Abilities.* Dissertation thesis. University of Detroit-Mercy.

Caron, J., and Lichtenberg, P.L. (1996 August). *Predictors of Geriatric Rehabilitation Patients' IADL Performance.* Paper presented at the annual meeting of the American Psychological Association, Toronto.

Charlson, M.E., Pompei, P., Ales, K.L., and MacKenzie, C.R. (1987). A new method of classifying prognostic comorbidity in longitudinal studies: Development and validation. *Journal of Chronic Diseases, 40*, 373-383.

Cockburn, J., Smith, P.T., and Wade, D.T. (1990). Influence of cognitive function on social, domestic and leisure activities of community-dwelling older people. *International Disability Studies, 12*, 169-172 .

Danielczyk, W. (1983). Various mental behavioral disorders in Parkinson's disease, primary degenerative senile dementia, and multiple infarction dementia. *Journal of Neural Transmission, 56*, 161-176.

Friedman, P.J. (1993). Stroke outcome in elderly people living alone. *Disability and Rehabilitation, 17*(2), 90-93.

Granger, C.V., Cotter, A.C., Hamilton, B.G., Roger, C.F., and Hens, M.M. (1990). Functional assessment scales: A study of persons with multiple sclerosis. *Archives of Physical Medicine and Rehabilitation, 71*, 870-875.

Green, J., Goldstein, F., Sirockman B., and Green, R. (1991). Variable awareness of deficits in Alzheimer's disease. *Neuropsychiatry, Neuropsychology, and Behavioral Neurology, 6*, 159-165.

Gustafson, L., and Nilsson, L. (1982). Differential diagnosis of presenile dementia on clinical grounds. *Acta Psychiatra Scandinavia, 65,* 194-209.

Hamilton, B.B., Laughlin, J.A., Granger, C.V., and Kayton, R.M. (1991). Interrater agreement of the seven level Functional Independence Measure (FIM). *Archives of Physical Medicine and Rehabilitation, 69,* 790.

Heilman, K. (1991). Anosognosia: Possible neuropsychological mechanisms. In G. Prigatano and D. Shacter (Eds.), *Awareness of Deficit After Brain Injury* (pp. 53-62). New York: Oxford University Press.

Isaac, L., and Tamblyn, R. (1993). Compliance and cognitive function: A methodological approach to measuring unintentional errors in medication compliance in the elderly. *The Gerontologist, 33,* 772-781.

Lawton, M.P., and Brody, E. (1969). Assessment of older people: Self-maintaining and instrumental activities of daily living. *The Gerontologist, 9,* 179-186.

Loewenstein, D.A., Rubert, M.P., Berkowitz-Zimmer, N., Guterman, A., Morgan, R., and Hayden, S. (1992). Neuropsychological test performance and prediction of functional capacities in dementia. *Behavior, Health, and Aging, 2*(3), 149-158.

MacNeill, S., and Lichtenberg, P.L. (in press). Home alone: The role of cognition in return to independent living. *Archives of Physical Rehabilitation.*

Mangone, C., Hier, D., Gorelick, P., Ganellen, R., Langenberg, P., Boarman, R., and Dollear, W. (1991). Impaired insight in Alzheimer's disease. *Journal of Geriatric Psychiatry and Neurology, 4,* 189-193.

Mahurin, R., DeBettignies, B., and Priozzolo, F. (1991). Structured assessment of independent living skills: Preliminary report of a performance measure of functional abilities in dementia. *Journal of Gerontology, 46*(2), 58-66.

Mattis, S. (1976). Mental status examination for organic mental syndromes in the elderly patient. In L. Beliak and T.B. Kraus (Eds.), *Geriatric Psychiatry.* New York: Oxford University Press.

McCue, M., Rogers, J.C., and Goldstein, G. (1990). Relationships between neuropsychology and functional assessment in elderly neuropsychiatric patients. *Rehabilitation Psychology, 35(2),* 91-99.

Moore, C.A. (1994). *The prediction of independent functioning through the use of selected neuropsychological tests.* Unpublished doctoral dissertation, Wayne State University, Detroit, MI.

Moore, C.A., and Lichtenberg, P.A. (1995). Neuropsychological prediction of independent functioning in a geriatric sample: A double cross validational study. *Rehabilitation Psychology, 41,* 115-130.

Nadler, J., Richardson, E.D., Malloy, P.F., Marran, M.E., and Brinson, M.E. (1993). The ability of the Dementia Rating Scale to predict everyday functioning. *Archives of Clinical Neuropsychology, 8,* 449-460.

Odenheimer, G.L., Beaudet, M., Jette, A.M., Albert, M.S., Grande, L., and Minaker, K.L. (1994). Performance-based driving evaluation of the elderly driver: Safety, reliability and validity. *Journal of Gerontology: Medical Sciences, 49,* 153-159.

Owsley, C., Ball, K., Sloane, M.E., Roenker, D.L., and Bruni, J.R. (1991). Visual/cognitive correlates of vehicle accidents in older drivers. *Psychology and Aging, 6,* 403-415.

Palmer, H.M. and Dobson, K.S. (1994). Self-medication and memory in an elderly Canadian sample. *The Gerontologist, 34*(5), 658-664.

Reisberg, B., Gordon, B., McCarthy, M., and Ferris, S. (1985). Clinical symptoms accompanying progressive cognitive decline and Alzheimer's disease. In V. Melnick and N. Dubler (Eds.), *Alzheimer's Dementia* (pp. 19-39). Clifton, NJ: Humana Press.

Reitan, R.M. (1955). Investigation of the validity of Halstead's measures of biological intelligence. *American Medical Association Archives of Neurology and Psychiatry, 73*, 28-35.

Richardson, E.D., Nadler, J.D., and Malloy, P.F. (1995). Neuropsychologic prediction of performance measures of daily living skills in geriatric patients. *Neuropsychology, 9*(4), 565-572.

Roth, E., Davidoff, G., Haughton, J., and Ardner, M. (1990). Functional assessment in spinal cord injury: A comparison of the modified Barthel Index and the "adapted" Functional Independence Measure. *Clinical Rehabilitation, 4*, 277-285.

Searight, H.R., Dunn, E.J., Grisso, T., Margolis, R.B., and Gibbons, J.L. (1989). The relation of the Halstead-Reitan Neuropsychological Battery to ratings of everyday functioning in a geriatric sample. *Neuropsychology, 3*, 135-145.

Titus, M., Gall, N., Yerxa, E., Roberson, T., and Mack, W. (1991). Correlation of perceptual performance and activities of daily living in stroke patients. *The American Journal of Occupational Therapy, 45*, 410-418.

Tuokko, H.A., and Crockett, D.J. (1991). Assessment of everyday functioning in normal and malignant memory-disordered elderly. In D.E. Tupper and K.D. Cicerone (Eds.), *The Neuropsychology of Everyday Life: Issues in Development and Rehabilitation* (135-182). Boston: Kluweer Academic Publishers.

Tupper, D.E., and Cicerone, K.D. (Eds.) (1990). *The Neuropsychology of Everyday Life: Assessment of Basic Competencies.* Boston: Kluweer Academic Publishers.

Tupper, D.E. and Cicerone, K.D. (Eds.) (1991). *The Neuropsychology of Everyday Life: Issues in Development and Rehabilitation.* Boston: Kluweer Academic Publishers.

Wagner, M.T., and Zuchigna, C.J. (1988). Longitudinal comparison of the Barthel and FIM during the first six months of recovery from stroke. *Archives of Physical Medicine and Rehabilitation, 69*, 775.

Wilking, S.V., Dowling, T.M., and Heeran, T. (1991). Correlations of Functional Independence Measure with Management Minutes Questionnaire on a special care Alzheimer unit. *Journal of the American Geriatrics Society, 39*(8), 76.

Wolinsky, F.D., Callahan, C.M., Fitzgerald, J.F., and Johnson, R.J. (1993). Changes in functional status and the risks of subsequent nursing home placement and death. *Journal of Gerontology: Social Sciences, 48*, 93-101.

Chapter 3

Bacher, Y., Korner-Bitensky, N., Mayo, N., Becker, R., and Coopersmith, H. (1990). A longitudinal study of depression among stroke patients participating in a rehabilitation program. *Canadian Journal of Rehabilitation, 1*, 27-37.

Blazer, D., Hughes, D., and George, L. (1987). The epidemiology of depression in an elderly community population. *The Gerontologist, 27*, 281-287.

Brink, T., Yesavage, J., Lum, G., Heersema, P., Addey, M., and Rose, T. (1982) Screening tests for geriatric depression. *Clinical Gerontologist, 1*, 37-41.

Brown, W.F. (1974). Effectiveness of paraprofessionals: The evidence. *Personnel and Guidance Journal, 53*, 257-263.

Cummings, S., Phillips, S., Wheat, M., Black, D., Goosby, E., Wlodarcyzk, D., Trafton, P., Jergesen, H., Winograd, C., and Hulley, S. (1988). Recovery of function after hip fracture: The role of social supports. *Journal of the American Geriatrics Society, 36*, 801-806.

Diamond, P.T., Holroyd, S., Macciocchi, S.N., and Felsenthal, G. (1995). Prevalence of depression and outcome on the geriatric rehabilitation unit. *American Journal of Physical Medicine and Rehabilitation, 74*, 214-217.

Durlak, J.A. (1979). Comparative effectiveness of paraprofessional and professional helpers. *Psychological Bulletin, 86*, 80-92.

Hanks, R.A., and Lichtenberg, P.A. (1996). Physical, psychological and social outcomes in geriatric rehabilitation patients. *Archives of Physical Medicine and Rehabilitation, 77*, 783-792.

Kafonek, S., Ettinger, W.H., Roca, R., Kittner, S., Taylor, N., and German, P.S. (1989). Instruments for screening for depression and dementia in a long-term care facility. *Journal of the American Geriatrics Society, 37*, 29-34.

Kanner, A., Coyne, J., Schaefer, C., and Lazarus, R. (1981). Comparison of two modes of stress management: Daily hassles and uplifts versus major life events. *Journal of Behavioral Medicine, 4*, 1-39.

Kitchell, M.A., Barnes, R.F., Veith, R.C., Okimoto, J.T., and Raskind, M.A. (1982). Screening for depression in hospitalized geriatric medical patients. *Journal of the American Geriatrics Society, 30*, 174-177.

Kramer, M., German, P., Anthony, J., Von Korff, M., and Skinner, E. (1985). Patterns of mental disorders among the elderly residents of eastern Baltimore. *Journal of the American Geriatrics Society, 33*, 236-245.

Lewinsohn, P.M., and Graf, M. (1973). Pleasant activities and depression. *Journal of Consulting and Clinical Psychology, 41*, 261-268.

Lewinsohn, P., and Talkington, J. (1979). Studies in the measurement of unpleasant life events and relations with depression. *Applied Psychological Measurement, 3*, 83-101.

Lichtenberg, P.A. (1994). *A Guide to Psychological Practice in Geriatric Long-Term Care*. Binghamton, NY: The Haworth Press.

Lichtenberg, P.A., and Barth, J.T. (1990). Depression in elderly caregivers: A longitudinal study to test Lewinsohn's model of depression. *Medical Psychotherapy, 3*, 147-156.

Lichtenberg, P.A., Christensen, B., Metler, L., Nanna, M., Jones, G., Reyes, J., and Blumenthal, F. (1994). A preliminary investigation of the role of cognition and depression in predicting functional recovery in geriatric rehabilitation patients. *Advances in Medical Psychotherapy, 7*, 109-124.

Lichtenberg, P.A., Gibbons, T.A., Nanna, M., and Blumenthal, F. (1993). Physician detection of depression in medically ill elderly. *Clinical Gerontologist, 13(1),* 81-90.

Lichtenberg, P.A., Marcopulos, B.A., Steiner, D., and Tabscott, J. (1992). Comparison of the Hamilton Depression Rating Scale and the Geriatric Depression Scale: Detection of depression in dementia patients. *Psychological Reports, 70,* 515-521.

Lichtenberg, P.A., Swensen, C.H., and Skehan, M.W. (1986). Further investigation of the role of personality, lifestyle and arthritic severity in predicting pain. *Journal of Psychosomatic Research, 30,* 327-337.

Livingston Bruce, M.L., Seeman, T.E., Merrill, S.S., and Blazer, D.G. (1994). The impact of depressive symptomatology on physical disability: MacArthur studies on successful aging. *American Journal of Public Health, 84,* 1796-1799.

Magaziner, J., Simonsick, E.M., Kashner, T.M., Hebel, J.R., and Kenzora, J.E. (1990). Predictors of functional recovery one year following hospital discharge for hip fracture. *Journal of Gerontology, 45,* M101-107.

Mattis, S. (1988). *Dementia Rating Scale: Professional Manual.* Odessa, FL: Psychological Assessment Resources.

Moore, J.T., Silimperi, D.R., and Bobula, J.A. (1978). Recognition of depression by family medicine residents: The impact of screening. *Journal of Family Practice, 7,* 509-513.

Nielsen, A.C., and Williams, T.A. (1980). Depression in ambulatory medical patients: Prevalence by self-report questionnaire and recognition by nonpsychiatric physicians. *Archives of General Psychiatry, 37,* 999-1004.

Norris, J.T., Gallagher, D., Wilson, A., and Winograd, C.H. (1987). Assessment of depression in geriatric medical outpatients: The validity of two screening measures. *Journal of the American Geriatrics Society, 35,* 989-995.

Okimoto, J.T., Barnes, R.F., Veith, R.C., Raskind, M.A., Inui, T.S., and Carter, W.B. (1982). Screening for depression in geriatric medical patients. *American Journal of Psychiatry, 139,* 799-802.

Parikh, R., Robinson, R., Lipsey, J., Starkstein, S., Federoff, J. and Price, T. (1990). The impact of poststroke depression on recovery in activities of daily living. *Archives of Neurology, 47,* 785-789.

Parmelee, P.A., Katz, I.R., and Lawton, M.P. (1989). Depression among institutionalized aged: Assessment and prevalence estimation. *Journal of Gerontology, 44,* M22-M29.

Primeau, F. (1988). Post-stroke depression: A critical review of the literature. *Canadian Journal of Psychiatry, 33,* 757-765.

Rapp, S.R., Parisi, S.A., Walsh, D.A., and Wallace, C.E. (1988). Detecting depression in elderly medical inpatients. *Journal of Consulting and Clinical Psychology, 56,* 509-513.

Rapp, S.R., Parisi, S.A., and Walsh, D.A. (1988). Psychological dysfunction and physical health among elderly medical inpatients. *Journal of Consulting and Clinical Psychology, 56,* 851-855.

Rattenbury, C., and Stones, M.J. (1989). A controlled evaluation of reminiscence and current topics discussion groups in a nursing home context. *The Gerontologist, 29*, 768-771.

Schuckit, M.A., Miller, P.L., and Halbohn, D. (1975). Unrecognized psychiatric illness in elderly medical-surgical patients. *Journal of Gerontology, 60*, 655-660.

Scogin, F., and McElreath, L. (1994). Efficacy of psychosocial treatments for geriatric depression: A quantitative review. *Journal of Consulting and Clinical Psychology, 62*, 69-74.

Shay, K.A., Duke, L., Conboy, T., Harrell, L., Callaway, R., and Folks, D.G. (1991). The clinical validity of the Mattis Dementia Rating Scale in the staging of Alzheimer's disease. *Journal of Geriatric Psychiatry and Neurology, 4*, 18-25.

Spitzer, R.L., and Endicott, J. (1979). *Schedule of Affective Disorders and Schizophrenia*. New York: New York State Psychiatric Institute.

Teri, L., and Gallagher-Thompson, D. (1991). Cognitive-behavioral interventions for treatment of depression in Alzheimer patients. *The Gerontologist, 31*, 413-416.

Teri, L., and Lewinsohn, P. (1982). Modification of the pleasant and unpleasant events schedules for use with the elderly. *Journal of Consulting and Clinical Psychology, 50*, 444-445.

Teri, L., and Logsdon, R.G. (1991). Identifying pleasant activities for Alzheimer disease patients: The Pleasant Events Schedule-AD. *The Gerontologist, 31*, 124-127.

Teri, L., and Uomoto, J.M. (1991). Reducing excess disability in dementia patients: Training caregivers to manage patient depression. *Clinical Gerontologist, 10*, 49-63.

Thompson, L. W., Gallagher, D., and Breckenridge, J.S. (1987). Comparative effectiveness of psychotherapies for depressed elders. *Journal of Consulting and Clinical Psychology, 55*, 385-390.

Waxman, H.M., and Carner, E.A. (1984). Physicians' Recognition, Diagnosis, and Treatment of Mental Disorders in Elderly Medical Patients. *The Gerontologist, 24*, 593-597.

Yesavage, J., Brink, T., Rose, T., Lum, O., Huang, V., Adez, M., Leirer, V. (1983). Development and validation of a Geriatric Depression Screening Scale: A preliminary report. *Journal of Psychiatric Research, 17*, 37-49.

Chapter 4

Albert, M.S. (1981). Geriatric neuropsychology. *Journal of Consulting and Clinical Psychology, 49*, 835-850.

Becker, J.T., Boller, F., Lopez, O.L., Saxton, J., and McGonigle, K.L. (1994). The natural history of Alzheimer's disease: Description of study cohort on accuracy of diagnosis. *Archives of Neurology, 51*, 585-594.

Christensen, H., Hadzi-Pavlovic, D., and Jacomb, P. (1991). The psychometric differentiation of dementia from normal aging: A meta-analysis. *Psychological Assessment: Journal of Consulting and Clinical Psychology, 3*, 147-155.

Eslinger, P.J., Damasio, A.R., Benton, A.L., and Van Allen, M. (1985). Neurop-sychological detection of abnormal mental decline in older persons. *Journal of the American Medical Association, 253,* 670-674.

Heaton, R.K., Grant, I., and Matthews, C.G. (1991). *Comprehensive Norms for an Extended Halstead-Reitan Battery.* Odessa, FL: Psychological Assessment Resources.

Inouye, S.K., Albert, M.S., Mohs, R., Sun, K., and Berkman, L.F. (1993). Cognitive performance in high functioning community dwelling elderly population. *Journal of Gerontology: Medical Sciences, 48,* 146-151.

Ivnik, R.J., Malec, J.F., Tangalos, E.G., Petersen, R.C., Kokmen, E., and Kurland, L.T. (1992). Mayo's Older American Normative Studies: WMS-R Norms for ages 56-94. *The Clinical Neuropsychologist, 6(supplement),* 49-82.

Linn, R.T., Wolf, P.A., Bachman, D.L., Knoefel, J.E., Cobb, J.L., Belanger, A.J., Kaplan, E.F., and D'Agostino, R.B. (1995). The "preclinical phase" of probable Alzheimer's disease. *Archives of Neurology, 52,* 485-490.

Masur, D.M., Sliwinski, M., Lipton, R.B., Blau, A.D., and Crystal, H.A. (1994). Neuropsychological prediction of dementia and the absence of dementia in healthy elderly persons. *Neurology, 44,* 1427-1432.

Morris, J.C., Heyman, A., Mohs, R.C., Hughes, J.P., van Belle, G., Fillenbaum, G., Mellits, E.D., and Clark, C. (1989). Consortium to establish a registry for Alzheimer's disease (CERAD). *Neurology, 39,* 1159-1165.

Petersen, R.C., Smith, G.E., Ivnik, R.J., Kokmen, E., and Tangalos, E.G., (1994). Memory function in very early Alzheimer's disease. *Neurology, 44,* 867-872.

Pincus, T., and Callahan, L.F. (1995). What explains the association between socioeconomic status and health: Primarily access to medical care or mind-body variables? *Advances: The Journal of Mind-Body Health, 11*(1), 4-36.

Robinson-Whelen, S., and Storandt, M. (1992). Immediate and delayed prose recall among normal and demented adults. *Archives of Neurology, 49,* 32-34.

Schaie, K.W. (1994). The course of adult intellectual development. *American Psychologist, 49,* 304-313.

Siegler, I.C., and Botwinick, J. (1979). A long-term longitudinal study of intellectual ability of older adults: The matter of selective subject attrition. *Journal of Gerontology, 34*(2), 242-245.

Spreen, O., and Strauss, E. (1991). *A Compendium of Neuropsychological Tests: Administration, Norms, and Commentary.* New York: Oxford University Press.

Storandt, M., Botwinick, J., and Danziger, W.L. (1986). Longitudinal changes: Patients with mild SDAT and matched healthy controls. In L.W. Poon (Ed.), *Handbook for clinical memory assessment of older adults* (pp. 277-284). Washington, DC: American Psychological Association.

Tarter, R. E., Van Thiel, D.H., and Edwards, K.L. (1988). *Medical neuropsychology.* New York: Plenum Press.

Taylor, J.L., Miller, T.P., and Tinkenberg, J.R. (1992). Correlates of memory decline: A 4-year longitudinal study of older adults with memory complaints. *Psychology and Aging, 7,* 183-193.

Unverzagt, F.W., Hall, K.S., Torke, A.M., Rediger, J.D., Mercado, N., Gureje, O., Osuntokun, B.O., and Hendrie, H.C. (1996). Effects of age, education and gender on CERAD neuropsychological test performance in an African American sample. *The Clinical Neuropsychologist, 10,* 180-190.

Verhaeghen, P., Marcoen, A., and Goossens, L. (1993). Facts and fiction about memory aging: A quantitative integration of research findings. *Journal of Gerontology: Psychological Sciences, 48,* P157-171.

Welsh, K., Butters, N., Hughes, J., Mohs, R., and Heyman, A. (1991). Detection of abnormal memory decline in mild cases of AD using CERAD neuropsychological measures. *Archives of Neurology, 48,* 278-281.

Welsh, K.A., Welsh, K.A., Butters, N., Mohs, R.C., Beckly, D., Edland, S., Fillenbaum, G., and Heyman, A. (1994). CERAD: A normative study of the neuropsychological battery. *Neurology, 44,* 609-614.

Youngjohn, J.R. and Crook, T.H. (1993). Learning, forgetting, and retrieval of everyday material across the lifespan. *Journal of Clinical and Experimental Neuropsychology, 15,* 447-460.

Chapter 5

Albert, M.S., Heller, H.S., and Milberg, W. (1988). Changes in naming ability with age. *Psychology and Aging, 3,* 173-178.

Benton, A.L., Hamsher, K., Varney, N.R., and Spreen, O. (1983). *Contributions to Neuropsychological Assessment.* New York: Oxford University Press.

Blair, J.R., and Spreen, O. (1989). Predicting premorbid IQ: A revision of the National Adult Reading Test. *Clinical Neuropsychologist, 3,* 129-136.

Boyd, J.L. (1981). A validity study of the Hooper Visual Organization Test. *Journal of Consulting and Clinical Psychology, 1,* 15-19.

Butters, N., Salmon, D.P., Cullum, C.M., Cairns, P., Troster, A.I., Jacobs, D., Moss, M., and Cermak, L.S. (1988). Differentiation of amnesic and demented patients with the Wechsler Memory Scale-Revised. *The Clinical Neuropsychologist, 2,* 133-148.

Coblentz, J.M., Mattis, S., Zingesser, L., Kasoff, S.S., Wisniewski, H.M., and Katzman, R. (1973). Presenile dementia: Clinical aspects and evaluation of cerebrospinal fluid dynamics. *Archives of Neurology, 29,* 299-308.

Cullum, C.M., Butters, N., Troster, A.I., and Salmon, D.P. (1990). Normal aging and forgetting rates on the Wechsler Memory Scale-Revised. *Archives of Clinical Neuropsychology, 5,* 23-30.

Christensen, H., Pavlovic-Hadzi, D., and Jacomb, P. (1992). The psychometric differentiation of dementia from normal aging: A meta-analysis. *Psychological Assessment: A Journal of Consulting and Clinical Psychology, 2,* 147-155.

Fuld, P.A. (1977). *Fuld Object Memory Evaluation.* New York: Albert Einstein College of Medicine.

Fuld, P.A. (1980). Guaranteed stimulus processing in the evaluation of memory and learning. *Cortex, 16,* 255-271.

Gardner, R., Oliver-Muñoz, S., Fisher, L., and Empting, L. (1981). Mattis Dementia Rating Scale: Internal reliability study using a diffusely impaired population. *Journal of Clinical Neuropsychology, 3*, 271-275.

Gerson, A. (1974). Validity and reliability of the Hooper Visual Organization Test. *Perceptual and Motor Skills, 39*, 95-100.

Heilman, K. M., and Valenstein, E. (Eds.) (1993). *Clinical Neuropsychology* Third Edition. New York: Oxford University Press.

Hooper, H. (1958). *The Hooper Visual Organization Test*. Los Angeles: Western Psychological Services.

Ivnik, R.J., Malec, J.F., Tangalos, E.G., Petersen, R.C., Kokmen, E., and Kurland, L.T. (1992). Mayo's older American normative studies: WMS-R norms for ages 56 to 94. *The Clinical Neuropsychologist, 6* (supplement), 49-82.

Kaplan, E., Goodglass, H., and Weintraub, S. (1978). *The Boston Naming Test*. Boston: E. Kaplan and H. Goodglass.

Kaplan, E., Goodglass, H., and Weintraub, S. (1983) *Boston Naming Test*. Philadelphia: Lea and Febiger.

Kimbarow, M.L., Vangel, S.J. and Lichtenberg, P.A. (1996). The influence of demographic variables on normal elderly adults' performance on the Boston Naming Test. *Clinical Aphasiology, 24*, 135-144.

LaBarge, E., Edwards, D., and Knesevich, J.W. (1986) Performance of normal elderly on the Boston Naming Test. *Brain and Language, 27*, 380-384.

LaRue, A. (1989). Patterns of performance on the Fuld Object Memory Evaluation in elderly inpatients with depression or dementia. *Journal of Clinical and Experimental Neuropsychology, 11*, 409-422.

LaRue, A., D'Elia, L., Clark, E., Spar, J., and Jarvik, L. (1986). Clinical tests of memory in dementia, depression and healthy aging. *Journal of Psychology and Aging, 1*, 69-77.

Libon, D.J., Glosser, G., Malamut, B.L., Kaplan, E., Goldberg, E., Swenson, R., and Sands, L.P. (1994). Age, executive functions, and visuospatial functioning in healthy older adults. *Neuropsychology, 8*, 38-43.

Lichtenberg, P.A., and Christensen, B. (1992). Extended normative data for the logical memory subtests of the Wechsler Memory Scale-Revised: Responses from a sample of cognitively intact elderly medical patients. *Psychological Reports, 71*, 745-746.

Lichtenberg, P.A., Millis, S.R., and Nanna, M. (1994). Use of Visual Form Discrimination Test with geriatric urban medical inpatients. *The Clinical Neuropsychologist, 8*, 462-465.

Lichtenberg, P.A., Ross, T., and Christensen, B. (1994). Preliminary normative data on the Boston Naming Test for an older urban population. *The Clinical Neuropsychologist, 8*, 109-111.

Lichtenberg, P.A., Ross, T.P., Youngblade, L., and Vangel, S.J. (n.d.). Normative Studies Research Project Test Battery.

Lichtenberg, P.A., Vangel, S.J., Kimbarow, M.L., and Ross, T.P. (1996). Clinical utility of the Boston Naming Test. *Clinical Gerontologist, 16*, 69-72.

Love, H.G. (1970). Validation of the Hooper Visual Organization Test on a New Zealand psychiatric hospital population. *Psychological Reports, 27*, 915-917.

Masur, D.M., Sliwinski, M., Lipton, R.B., Blau, A.D., and Crystal, H.A. (1994). Neuropsychological prediction of dementia and the absence of dementia in healthy elderly persons. *Neurology, 44,* 1427-1432.

Mattis, S. (1988). *Dementia Rating Scale: Professional Manual.* Odessa, FL: Psychological Assessment Resources.

Mitrushina, M., and Satz, P. (1989) Differential decline of specific memory components in normal aging. *Brain Dysfunction, 2,* 330-335.

Montgomery, K.M., and Costa, L. (1983). *Neuropsychological Test Performance of a Normal Elderly Sample.* Presented at International Neuropsychological Society meeting, Mexico City, Mexico.

Moses, J.A. (1986). Factor structure of Benton's tests of Visual Retention, Visual Construction and Visual Form Discrimination. *Archives of Clinical Neuropsychology, 1,* 147-156.

Moses, J.A. (1989). Replicated factor structure of Benton's tests of Visual Retention, Visual Construction and Visual Form Discrimination. *International Journal of Clinical Neuropsychology, 11,* 30-37.

Nabors, N.A., Vangel, S.J., and Lichtenberg, P.A. (1996). Normative data and clinical utility of the Visual Form Discrimination Test with geriatric medical inpatients. *Clinical Gerontologist, 17,* 43-53.

Nabors, N.A., Vangel, S.J., Lichtenberg, P.A., and Walsh, P. (in press). Normative and clinical utility of the Hooper Visual Organization Test with geriatric medical inpatients. *Journal of Clinical Geropsychology.*

Nicholas, M., Obler, L., Albert, M., and Goodglass, H. (1985). Lexical retrieval in healthy aging. *Cortex, 21,* 595-606.

Paque, L., and Warrington, E.K. (1995). A longitudinal study of reading ability in patients suffering from dementia. *Journal of the International Neuropsychological Society, 1,* 517-524.

Ross, T.P., Lichtenberg, P.A., and Christensen, B.K. (1995). Normative data on the Boston Naming Test for elderly adults in a demographically diverse medical sample. *The Clinical Neuropsychologist, 9,* 321-325.

Ryan, J.J., and Paolo, A.M. (1992). A screening procedure for estimating premorbid intelligence in the elderly. *The Clinical Neuropsychologist, 6*(1), 53-62.

Schmidt, R., Freidl, W., Fazekas, F., Reinhart, P., Grieshofer, P., Koch, M., Eber, B., Schumacher, M., Polmin, K., and Lechner, H. (1994). The Mattis Dementia Rating Scale: Normative data from 1,001 healthy volunteers. *Neurology, 44,* 964-966.

Shay, K., Duke, L., Conboy, T., Harrell, L.E., Callaway, R., and Folks, D.G. (1991). The clinical validity of the Mattis Dementia Rating Scale in staging Alzheimer's dementia. *Journal of Geriatric Psychiatry and Neurology, 4,* 18-25.

Summers, J.D., Lichtenberg, P.A., and Vangel, S.J. (1995). Normative and discriminability properties of the Fuld Object Memory Evaluation in an urban geriatric population. *Clinical Gerontologist, 15,* 21-34.

Troster, A.I., Butters, N., Salmon, D.P., Cullum, C.M., Jacobs, D., Brandt, J., and White, R.F. (1993). The diagnostic utility of savings scores: Differentiating Alzheimer's and Huntington's diseases with the Logical Memory and Visual Reproduction Tests. *Journal of Clinical and Experimental Neuropsychology, 15*(5), 773-788.

Vangel, S.J., Lichtenberg, P.A., and Ross, T.P. (in press). Clinical utility of the logical memory subtest and the relationship of demographic factors to test performance. *Journal of Clinical Geropsychology.*

Vangel, S.J., and Lichtenberg, P.A. (1995). The Mattis Dementia Rating Scale: Clinical utility and relationship with demographic variables. *The Clinical Neuropsychologist, 9*, 209-213.

VanGorp, W.G., Satz, P., Evans-Kiersch, M., and Henry, R. (1986). Normative data on the Boston Naming Test for a Group of Normal Older Adults. *Journal of Clinical and Experimental Neuropsychology, 8*, 702-705.

Vitaliano, P.P., Breen, A.R., Russo, J., Albert, M.S., Vitiello, M., and Prinz, P.N. (1984). The clinical utility of the Dementia Rating Scale for assessing Alzheimer's patients. *Journal of Chronic Disabilities, 37*(9/10), 743-753.

Walsh, P.F., Lichtenberg, P.A., and Rowe, R.J. (1997). Hooper Visual Organization Test performance in geriatric rehabilitation patients. *Clinical Gerontologist, 17,* 3-13.

Wechsler, D. (1987). *The Wechsler Memory Scale-Revised.* New York: Psychological Corporation.

Wiens, A.N., Bryan, J.E., and Crossen, J.R. (1993). Estimating WAIS-R FSIQ from the National Adult Reading Test-Revised in normal subjects. *The Clinical Neuropsychologist, 7*(1), 70-84.

Chapter 6

Albert, M.S., Levkoff, S.E., Reilly, C., Liptzin, B., Pilgrim, D., Cleary, P.D., Evens, D., and Rowe, J.W. (1992). The delirium symptom interview: An interview for the detection of delirium symptoms in hospitalized patients. *Journal of Geriatric Psychiatry and Neurology, 5*, 14-21.

Albert, M.L., and Knoefel, J.E. (Eds.) (1994). *Clinical Neurology of Aging,* Second Edition. New York: Oxford University Press.

Cummings, J.L. (1993). The neuroanatomy of depression. *Journal of Clinical Psychiatry, 54*(11), 14-20.

Hanks, R.A., and Lichtenberg, P.A. (1996). Physical, psychological and social outcomes in geriatric rehabilitation patients. *Archives of Physical Medicine and Rehabilitation, 77,* 783-792.

LaRue, A. (1993). *Aging and Neuropsychological Assessment.* New York: Plenum Press.

Lichtenberg, P.A. (1994). *A Guide to Psychological Practice in Geriatric Long-Term Care.* Binghamton, NY: The Haworth Press.

Malec, J.F., Smith, G.E., Ivnik, R.J., Petersen, R.C., and Tangalos, E.G. (1996). Clusters of impaired normal elderly do not decline cognitively in 3 to 5 years. *Neuropsychology, 10*(1), 66-73.

Meneilly, G.S., Cheung, E., Tessier, D., Yakura, C., and Tuokko, H. (1993). The effect of improved glycemic control on cognitive functions in the elderly patient with diabetes. *Journal of Gerontology, 48*(4), M117-M121.

Millis, S.R. (1992). The Recognition Memory Test in the detection of malingered and exaggerated memory deficits. *The Clinical Neuropsychologist, 6*(4), 406-414.

Millis, S.R. (1994). Assessment of motivation and memory with the Recognition Memory Test after financially compensable mild head injury. *Journal of Clinical Psychology, 50*(4), 601-605.

Rockwood, K. (1993). The occurrence and duration of symptoms in elderly patients with delirium. *Journal of Gerontology: Medical Sciences, 48*, 162-166.

Ryan, C., and Butters, N. (1986). The neuropsychology of alcoholism. In D. Wedding, A. Horton, and J. Webster (Eds.) *The Neuropsychology Handbook.* New York: Springer, 376-409.

Salerno, J.A., Grady, C., Mentis, M., Gonzalez-Aviles, A., Wagner, E., Schapiro, M.B., and Rapoport, S.I. (1995). Brain metabolic function in older men with chronic essential hypertension. *Journal of Gerontology, 50A*(3), M147-M154.

Trzepacz, P.T., Baker, R.W., and Greenhouse, J. (1987). A symptom rating scale for delirium. *Psychiatry Research, 23*, 89-97.

Chapter 7

Blanchard, E.B., and Andrasik, F. (1985). *Management of Chronic Headaches: A Psychological Approach.* New York: Pergamon.

Brink, T., Yesavage, J., Lum, G., Heersema, P., Addey, M., and Rose, T. (1982). Screening tests for geriatric depression. *Clinical Gerontologist, 1*, 37-41.

Lewinsohn, P.M., Hoberman, H.M., and Clark, G.N. (1989). The coping with depression course: Review and future directions. *Canadian Journal of Behavioral Science, 21*, 470-493.

Lewinsohn, P., and Talkington, J. (1979). Studies in the measurement of unpleasant life events and relations with depression. *Applied Psychological Measurement, 3*, 83-101.

Phillips, H. C. (1988). *The Psychological Management of Chronic Pain: A Treatment Manual.* New York: Springer.

Teri, L., and Logsdon, R.G. (1991). Identifying pleasant activities for Alzheimer disease patients: The Pleasant Events Schedule-AD. *The Gerontologist, 31*, 124-127.

Teri, L., and Uomoto, J.M. (1991). Reducing excess disability in dementia patients: Training caregivers to manage patient depression. *Clinical Gerontologist, 10*, 49-63.

Chapter 8

Atkinson, R.M. and Ganzini, L. (1994). Substance abuse. In C.E. Coffey and J.L. Cummings (Eds.). *Textbook of geriatric neuropsychiatry.* Washington, DC: American Psychiatric Press, Inc., 298-321.

Atkinson, R.M. and Kofoed, L.L. (1982). Alcohol and drug abuse in old age: A clinical perspective. *Substance and Alcohol Actions/Misuse*, *3*, 353-368.

Benshoff, J.J., and Roberto, K.A. (1987). Alcoholism in the elderly: Clinical issues. *Clinical Gerontologist*, *7*, 3-15.

Beresford, T.P., Blow, F.C., Brower, K.J., Adams, K.M., and Hall, R.C. (1988). Alcoholism and aging in the general hospital. *Psychosomatics*, *29*, 61-72.

Brody, J.A. (1982). Aging and alcohol abuse. *Journal of the American Geriatrics Society*, *30*, 123-126.

Bush, B., Shaw, S., Cleary, P., Delbanco, T.L., and Aronson, M.D. (1987). Screening for alcohol abuse using the CAGE questionaire. *The American Journal of Medicine*, *82*, 231-235.

Curtis, J.R., Geller, G., Stokes, E., Levine, D.M., and Moore, R.D (1989). Characteristics, diagnosis, and treatment of alcoholism in elderly patients. *Journal of the American Geriatrics Society*, *37*, 310-316.

Diagnostic and Statistical Manual of Mental Disorders, Fourth Edition. (1994). Washington DC: American Psychiatric Association Press, Inc.

Donahue, R.P., Abbott, R.D., Reed, D.M., and Yano, K. (1986). Alcohol and hemorrhagic stroke: The Honolulu Heart Program. *Journal of the American Medical Association*, *255*(17), 2311-2314.

Douglass, R. (1984). Aging and alcohol problems: Opportunities for socioepidemiological research. In M. Galanter (Ed.), *Recent Developments in Alcoholism* (pp. 214-240). New York: Plenum Press.

Dupree, L.W., Broskowski, H., and Schonfeld, L. (1984). The gerontology alcohol project: A behavioral treatment program for elderly alcohol abusers. *The Gerontologist*, *24*, 510-516.

Eckardt, M.J. and Martin, P.R. (1986). Clinical assessment of cognition in alcoholism. *Alcoholism: Clinical and Experimental Research*, *10*, 123-127.

Ewing, J.A. (1984). Detecting alcoholism: The CAGE questionnaire. *Journal of the American Medical Association*, *252*, 1905-1907.

Goldstein, F.C. and Levin, H.S. (1987). Disorders of reasoning and problem solving ability. In M. Meier, A. Benton, and L. Diller (Eds.), *Neuropsychological Rehabilitation* (pp. 103-130). New York: Guilford Press.

Gomberg, E. (1990). Drugs, alcohol and aging. *Research Advances in Alcohol and Drug Problems*, *10*, 171-213.

Hanks, R.A. and Lichtenberg, P.A. (1996). Physical, psychological and social outcomes in geriatric rehabilitation patients. *Archives of Physical Medicine and Rehabilitation*.

Hartford, J. R. and Damorajski, T. (1982). Alcoholism in the geriatric population. *Journal of the American Geriatric Society*, *30*, 18.

Haut, M.J. and Cowan, D.H. (1974). The effect of ethanol on hemostatic properties of human blood platelets. *American Journal of Medicine*, *56*, 22-23.

Hedlund, J.L. and Vieweg, B.W. (1984). The Michigan alcoholism screening test (MAST): A comprehensive review. *Journal of Operational Psychiatry*, *15*, 55-64.

Hubbard, R.W., Santos, J.F., and Santos, M.A. (1979). Alcohol and older adults: Overt and covert influences. *Journal of Contemporary Social Work, March,* 166-170.

Janik, S.W. and Dunham, R.G. (1983). A nationwide examination of the need for specific alcoholism treatment programs for the elderly. *Journal of Studies on Alcohol, 44,* 307-317.

Johnson, L.K. (1989). How to diagnose and treat chemical dependency in the elderly. *Journal of Gerontological Nursing, 15*(12), 22-26.

Kofoed, L.L., Tolson, R.L., Atkinson, R.M., Roth, R.L., and Turner, J.A. (1987). Treatment compliance of older alcoholics: and elder-specific approach is superior to "Mainstreaming." *Journal of Studies on Alcohol, 48,* 47-51.

Larson, E.B., Reifler, B.V., and Sumi, S.M.. (1985). Diagnostic evaluation of 200 elderly outpatients with suspected dementia. *Journal of Gerontology, 40,* 536-543.

Liberto, J.G., Oslin, J.W., and Ruskin, P.E. (1992). Alcoholism in older persons: A review of the literature. *Hospital Community Psychiatry, 43,* 975-984.

Lichtenberg, P.A., Gibbons, T.A., Nanna, M.J., and Blumenthal, F. (1993). The effects of age and gender on the prevalence and detection of alcohol abuse in elderly medical patients. *Clinical Gerontologist, 13*(3), 17-27.

Maletta, G.J. (1982). Alcoholism and the aged. In W. Pattison, and G. Kaufman (Eds.), *Encyclopedia Handbook of Alcoholism* (pp. 779-791). Gardner Press: New York.

Marcus, M.T. (1993). Alcohol and other drug abuse in elders. *Journal of ET Nursing, 20,* 106-110.

Myers, A.R., Hingson, R., Mucatel, M., and Goldman, E. (1982). Social and psychologic correlates of problem drinking in old age. *Journal of the American Geriatrics Society, 30,* 452-456.

Nordstrom, G. and Berglund, M. (1987). Aging and recovery from alcoholism. *British Journal of Psychiatry, 15,* 382-388.

Parker, E.S. and Noble, E.P. (1980). Alcohol and the aging process in social drinkers. *Journal of Studies in Alcohol, 41,* 170-178.

Porkorney, A., Miller, B., and Kaplan, H. (1972). The brief MAST: A shortened version of the Michigan Alcoholism Screening Test. *American Journal of Psychiatry, 129,* 342-345.

Rains, V.S. and Ditzler, T.F. (1993). Alcohol use disorders in cognitively impaired patients referred for geriatric assessment. *Journal of Addictive Diseases, 12*(1), 55-64.

Rains, V.S., Ditzler, T.F., Blanchette, P. (1989). Recognition of alcohol dependence in the elderly. *Journal of the American Geriatrics Society, 37,* 1204-1205.

Rosin, A.J. and Glatt, M.M. (1971). Alcohol excess in the elderly. *Quarterly Journal of Studies on Alcoholism, 32,* 53-59.

Ryan, C. and Butters, N. (1986). The neuropsychology of alcoholism. In D. Wedding, A. Horton, and J. Webster (Eds.) *The neuropsychology handbook* (pp. 376-409). New York: Springer.

Schuckit, M.A. (1977) Geriatric alcoholism and drug abuse. *Gerontologist, 17,* 168-174.

Schukit, M.A., Atkinson, J.H., Miller, P.L., and Berman, J. (1980). A three-year follow-up of elderly alcoholics. *Journal of Clinical Psychiatry, 41*, 412-416.

Schukit, M.A. and Pastor, P.A. (1978). The elderly as a unique population: Alcoholism. *Alcoholism: Clinical and Experimental Research, 2*, 31-38.

Scott, R.B. and Mitchell, M.C. (1988). Aging, alcohol and the liver. *Journal of the American Geriatrics Society, 36*, 255-265.

Selzer, M.L. (1971). The Michigan alcoholism screening test (MAST): The quest for a new diagnostic instrument. *American Journal of Psychiatry, 127*, 1653-1658.

Sherose, D. (1983). *Professional's Handbook on Geriatric Alcoholism*. Springfield, IL: Charles C Thomas Publishing.

Sumberg, D. (1985). Social work with elderly alcoholics: Some practical considerations. *Gerontological Social Work Practice in the Community: Journal of Gerontological Social Work, 8*, 169-181.

Tarter, R., Van Thiel, D., and Edwards, K. (Eds.) (1988). *Medical neuropsychology*. New York: Plenum Press.

Thienhaus, O.J. and Hartford, J.T. (1984). Alcoholism in the elderly. *Psychiatric Medicine, 2*, 27-41.

Ticehurst, S. (1990). Alcohol and the elderly. *Australian and New Zealand Journal of Psychiatry, 24*, 252-260.

Wattis, J.P. (1981). Alcohol problems in the elderly. *Journal of the American Geriatrics Society, 29*, 131-134.

Willenbring, M.L., Christensen, K.J., Spring, W.D., and Rasmussen, R. (1987). Alcoholism screening in the elderly. *Journal of the American Geriatrics Society, 35*, 864-869.

Willenbring, M.L. (1988). Organic mental disorders associated with heavy drinking and alcohol dependence. *Clinics in Geriatric Medicine, 4*, 869-887.

Wolf, P.A., Dawber, T.R., Thomas, H.E., and Kannel, W.B. (1978). Epidemiologic assessment of chronic atrial fibrillation and risk of stroke: The Framingham study. *Neurology, 28*, 973-977.

Zimberg, S. (1984). Diagnosis and management of the elderly alcoholic. In R. Atkinson (Ed.), *Alcohol and Drug Abuse* American Psychiatric Press: Washington, DC, 23-33.

Chapter 9

Abernathy, V. (1984). Compassion, control, and decisions about competency. *American Journal of Psychiatry, 141*(1), 53-57.

Alexander, M.P. (1988). Clinical determination of mental competence: A theory and a retrospective study. *Archives of Neurology, 45*, 23-26.

American Psychological Association. (1994). *Medicare guidelines for psychologists*. Washington, DC: APA Practice Directorate.

Appelbaum, P.S. and Grisso, T. (1988). Assessing patients' capacities to consent to treatment. *The New England Journal of Medicine, 319*(25), 1635-1638.

Barbee, J.G. and McLaulin, J.B. (1990). Anxiety disorders: Diagnosis and pharmacotherapy in the elderly. *Psychiatric Annals, 20*(8), 439-445.

Casten, R.J., Parmelee, P.A., Kleban, M.H., Lawton, M.P., and Katz, I.R. (1995). The relationships among anxiety, depression, and pain in a geriatric institutionalized sample. *Pain, 61,* 271-276.

Dale, J.A. and DeGood, D.E. (in press). The emerging role of the psychologist in pain management. *Advances in Medical Psychotherapy, 9,* 1-20.

DeGood, D.E., Buckelew, S.P., and Tait, R.C. (1985). Cognitive-somatic anxiety response patterning in chronic pain patients and nonpatients. *Journal of Consulting and Clinical Psychology, 53,* 137-138.

Drane, J.F. (1984). Competency to give an informed consent. *Journal of the American Medical Association, 252*(7), 925-927.

Ferrell, B.A., Ferrell, B.R., and Osterweil, D.A. (1990). Pain in the nursing home. *Journal of the American Geriatrics Society, 38,* 409-414.

Fitten, L.J., Lusky, R., and Hamann, C. (1990). Assessing treatment decision-making capacity in elderly nursing home residents. *Journal of the American Geriatrics Society, 38,* 1097-1104.

Fitten, L.J. and Waite, M.S. (1990). Impact of medical hospitalization on treatment decision-making capacity in the elderly. *Archives of Internal Medicine, 150,* 1717-1721.

Grisso, T. (1994). Clinical assessments for legal competence of older adults. In M. Storandt and G.R. VandenBos (Eds.), *Neuropsychological assessment of dementia and depression in older adults: A clinician's guide* (pp. 119-140). Washington, DC: American Psychological Association.

Gutheil, T.G. and Bursztayn, H. (1986). Clinicians' guidelines for assessing and presenting subtle forms of patient incompetence in legal settings. *American Journal of Psychiatry, 143*(8), 1020-1023.

Himmelfarb, S. and Murrell, S.A. (1984). Prevalence and correlates of anxiety symptoms in older adults. *Journal of Psychology, 116,* 159-167.

Iris, M.A. (1988). Guardianship and the elderly: A multi-perspective view of the decision-making process. *The Gerontologist, 28,* 39-45.

Keith, P.M. and Wacker, R.R. (1993). Implementation of recommended guardianship practices and outcomes of hearings for older persons. *The Gerontologist, 33,* 81-87.

Lavsky-Shulan, M., Wallace, R.B., Kohout, F.J., Lemke, J.H., Morris, M.C., and Smith, I.M. (1985). Prevalence and functional correlates of low back pain in the elderly: The Iowa 65+ rural health study. *Journal of the American Geriatrics Society, 33,* 23-28.

Lichtenberg, P.A., Skehan, M.W., and Swensen, C.H. (1984). The role of personality, recent life stress and arthritic severity in predicting pain. *Journal of Psychosomatic Research, 28,* 231-236.

Lichtenberg, P.A., Swensen, C.H., and Skehan, M.W. (1986). Further investigation of the role of personality, lifestyle and arthritic severity in predicting pain. *Journal of Psychosomatic Research, 30,* 327-337.

Marson, D.C., Chatterjee, A., Ingram, K.K., and Harrell, L.E. (1996). Toward a neurologic model of competency: Cognitive predictors of capacity to consent in Alzheimer's disease using three different legal standards. *Neurology, 46,* 666-672.

Marson, D.C., Cody, H.A., Ingram, K.K., and Harrell, L.E. (1995). Neuropsychologic predictors of competency in Alzheimer's disease using a rational reasons legal standard. *Archives of Neurology, 52*, 955-959.

Marson, D.C., Ingram, K.K., Cody, H.A., and Harrell, L.E. (1995). Assessing the competency of patients with Alzheimer's disease under different legal standards. *Archives of Neurology, 52*, 949-954.

Melzack, R. and Wall, P.D. (1965). Pain mechanism: A new theory. *Science, 150*, 971-979.

Moye, J. (1996). Theoretical frameworks for competency in cognitively impaired elderly adults. *Journal of Aging Studies, 10*(1), 27-42.

Oberle, K., Paul, P., Wry, J., and Grace, M. (1990). Pain, anxiety and analgesics: A comparative study of elderly and younger surgical patients. *Canadian Journal on Aging, 9*, 13-22.

Parmelee, P.A., Kleban, M.H., and Katz, I.R. (in press). Pain, depression and anxiety among frail older persons: The role of somatic symptoms. *Advances in Medical Psychotherapy, 9,* 33-54.

Physician's current procedural terminology (CPT). (1995). Chicago, IL: American Medical Association.

Pruchno, R.A., Smyer, M.A., Rose, M.S., Hartman-Stein, P.E., and Henderson-Laribee, D.L. (1995). Competence of long-term care residents to participate in decisions about their medical care: A brief, objective assessment. *The Gerontologist, 35*(5), 622-629.

Roth, L.H., Meisel, A., and Lidz, C.W. (1977). Tests of competency to consent to treatment *American Journal of Psychiatry, 134*(3), 279-284.

Chapter 10

Benton, A.L., Hamsher, K., Varney, N.R., and Spreen, O. (1994). *Contributions to Neuropsychological Assessment (2nd edition).* New York: Oxford University Press.

Brown, H.N. and Zimberg, N.E. (1982). Difficulties in the integration of psychological and medical practices. *American Journal of Psychiatry, 139*, 1576-1580.

Hanks, R.A., and Lichtenberg, P.A. (1996). Physical, psychological, and social outcomes in geriatric rehabilitation patients. *Archives of Physical Medicine and Rehabilitation, 77,* 783-792.

Lichtenberg, P.A. (1994). *A Guide to Psychological Practice in Geriatric Long-Term Care.* Binghamton, NY: The Haworth Press.

Morris, J.C., Heyman, A., Mohs, R.C., Hughes, J.P., van Belle, G., Fillenbaum, G., Mellits, E.D., and Clark, C. (1989). Consortium to establish a registry for Alzheimer's disease (CERAD). *Neurology, 39,* 1159-1165.

Qualls, S.H. and Czirr, R. (1988). Geriatric health teams: Classifying models of professional and team functioning. *The Gerontologist, 28,* 372-376.

Index

Page numbers followed by the letter "t" indicate tables.

Competency *(continued)*
scales, 157
Competency assessment research,
limitations in, 161-164
Complainer hypothesis, 165-166
Conceptualization, 161
Conflict resolution, 173-174
Confrontational naming, 58,161
Confronting alcohol abuse in older
adults, 151-153
Consortium to Establish a Registry
for Alzheimer's Disease
(CERAD). *See* CERAD
battery
Continuous Improvement, 3
Continuum of care, 178
Controlled breathing, 122-125
Controlled Oral Word Association
test, 63,113,116
Controlling use of alcohol, 136
Correlation, 31t,91
Corticol dementia, 27
Costa, L., 71,90
Cost-containment changes, 175
Cowan, D.H., 134
Crockett, D.J., 18
Crook, T.H., 55
Crossen, J.R., 92
Crossing Off Test, 61
Cross-sectional data, 53,54
Cross-sectional research, 53-55
Cullum, C.M., 75,77
Cummings, J.L., 113
Cummings, S., 40
Curtis, J.R., 133,138,141,142
Czirr, R., 172

Daily Hassles Scale, 45
Daily mood ratings, 45
Dale, J.A., 168
Damorajski, T., 139,140
Danielczyk, W., 28
Danziger, W.L., 61,62,63
DeBettignies, B., 28,29

Decision-making capacity,
determining, 155-158
Decision tree for neuropsychology
referral, 176t
Deficit, 27-28
DeGood, D.E., 166,167,168
Delerium, 156
and alcohol withdrawal, 136
assessment of, 110
and dementia, 13
Dementia, 107
diagnosis of etiology of, 146
NSRP test battery for, 114-115
subcortical, 28
vascular, 28
vs. normal aging, 57-60
Dementia to delirium, 13
Dementia Rating Scale (DRS),
26,42,68,70
and competency, 161
and the NSRP Test Battery,
93,96,97
Demographic data, influence of, 85
Demographic variable, 33
and Boston Naming Test, 83
and NSRP Test Battery, 97
and Visual Form Discrimination
Test, 89
Depression, *xi*,1,9,166,167. *See also*
DOUR Project; Geriatric
depression
and activities of daily living skills,
49,51t
behavioral theory of, 43-45
behavioral treatment of, 119-121
case examples, 130-132
controlled breathing, 122-125
imagery, 122-125
mood monitoring, 121-122
Pleasant Events Schedule,
125-128
reinforcement, 129
relaxation, 122-125
clinical implications of, 52
and cognition, 13

George, L., 8,37
Geriatric depression, 43-44. *See also*
    Depression
Geriatric Depression Scale (GDS),
    13,38,39-40,42,131
    use of in the DOUR project, 47,
    48,49,50t
Geriatric medical patient, 11
Geriatric medical rehabilitation
    program, 15
Gerontology Alcohol Project, 149
Gerson, A., 90
Giuliano, Tony, 27
Glatt, M.M, 139,140
Goldstein, F., 16,17,147
Goldstein, G., 28
Gomberg, E., 143
Goodglass, H., 82
Goosens, L., 55
Graf, M., 44
Granger, C.V., 19
Graphs, 131
Grant, I., 57
Green, J., 28
Green, R., 28
Greenhouse, J., 110
Grisso, T., 155,156,158,159
Group therapy, 148
*Guide to Psychological Practice
    in Geriatric Long-Term
    Care, A,* 3,179
Gustafson, L., 28
Gutheil, T.G., 158

Hadzi-Pavlovic, D., 58
Hahlbohn, D., 38
Halstead Reitan Neuropsychological
    Battery (HRNB), 17,61
Hamann, C., 158
Hamilton, B.B., 19
Hamsher, K., 87
Hanks, R.A., 8,11,38,139,175
Harrell, L.E., 159,160
Hartford, J.R., 130,139,143

Haut, M.J., 134
Health Care Financing
    Administration, 169
Health care provider, practice
    management issues, 169-170
Health care setting
    and detection of alcohol abuse,
    138
    and shaping referrals in, 174-178
Health outcome, and cognition,
    15-16
Health system, opportunities
    in, 178-179
Heaton, R.K., 57
Hedlund, J.L., 143
Heeran, T., 19
Heilman, K., 27,81
Heller, H.S., 82
Hertz, P., 3
Heteroskedasticity, 73
Himmelfarb, S., 164
Hirschon, B.A., 3
Hoberman, H.M., 121
Hooper, H., 90,91. *See also* Hooper
    Visual Organization Test
Hooper Visual Organization Test,
    90-91
    normative observations for older
    adults, 92t
    and the NSRP Test Battery, 93,96
    case illustrations, 113,116
Hopemont Capacity Assessment
    Inventory, 160
Hospitalization
    and discharge from, 20
    and length of stay, 20
    and loss of independence, 10
Hubbard, R.W., 144
Hughes, D., 8,37
Huntington's disease, 75
Hypochondriacal and Depression
    scale, 165

IADL. *See* Instrumental activities
    of daily living

Wells, C.E., 13
Welsh, K.A., 65
Wide Range Achievement Test—
    Revised (WRAT-R), 92
Wiens, A.N., 92
Wilking, S.V., 19
Willenbring, M.L., 137
Williams, T.A., 38
Withdrawal (alcohol), 134
    symptoms, 136
WMS-R. *See* Wechsler Memory
    Scale—Revised
Wolf, P.A., 134

Wolinsky, F.D., 25
WRAT-R. *See* Wide Range
    Achievement Test—Revised

Yesavage, J., 13,39
Young adult, and comorbid disease, 8
Youngjohn, J.R., 55

Zimberg, N.E., 171,172
Zimberg, S., 133,145,146
Zuchigna, C.J., 19

Order Your Own Copy of
This Important Book for Your Personal Library!

MENTAL HEALTH PRACTICE IN GERIATRIC HEALTH CARE SETTINGS

_____ in hardbound at $49.95 (ISBN: 0-7890-0117-9)

_____ in softbound at $24.95 (ISBN: 0-7890-0435-6)

COST OF BOOKS_____

OUTSIDE USA/CANADA/
MEXICO: ADD 20%_____

POSTAGE & HANDLING_____
(US: $3.00 for first book & $1.25
for each additional book)
Outside US: $4.75 for first book
& $1.75 for each additional book)

SUBTOTAL_____

IN CANADA: ADD 7% GST_____

STATE TAX_____
(NY, OH & MN residents, please
add appropriate local sales tax)

FINAL TOTAL_____
(If paying in Canadian funds,
convert using the current
exchange rate. UNESCO
coupons welcome.)

☐ **BILL ME LATER:** ($5 service charge will be added)
(Bill-me option is good on US/Canada/Mexico orders only;
not good to jobbers, wholesalers, or subscription agencies.)

☐ Check here if billing address is different from
shipping address and attach purchase order and
billing address information.

Signature_____

☐ **PAYMENT ENCLOSED: $**_____

☐ **PLEASE CHARGE TO MY CREDIT CARD.**

☐ Visa   ☐ MasterCard   ☐ AmEx   ☐ Discover
☐ Diner's Club

Account #_____

Exp. Date_____

Signature_____

Prices in US dollars and subject to change without notice.

NAME _____

INSTITUTION _____

ADDRESS _____

CITY _____

STATE/ZIP _____

COUNTRY _____ COUNTY (NY residents only) _____

TEL _____ FAX _____

E-MAIL_____
May we use your e-mail address for confirmations and other types of information? ☐ Yes   ☐ No

Order From Your Local Bookstore or Directly From
The Haworth Press, Inc.
10 Alice Street, Binghamton, New York 13904-1580 • USA
TELEPHONE: 1-800-HAWORTH (1-800-429-6784) / Outside US/Canada: (607) 722-5857
FAX: 1-800-895-0582 / Outside US/Canada: (607) 772-6362
E-mail: getinfo@haworth.com
PLEASE PHOTOCOPY THIS FORM FOR YOUR PERSONAL USE.

BOF96